T0176910

An Illustrated Guide to Oral Histology

An Illustrated Guide to Oral Histology

Edited by

Imran Farooq

BDS (Pak), MFGDP RCS (UK), MFDS RCPS (UK), MSc Oral Biology (UK)
Department of Biomedical Dental Sciences
College of Dentistry
Imam Abdulrahman Bin Faisal University
Dammam, Saudi Arabia

Saqib Ali

BDS (Pak), MFGDP RCS (UK), MFDS RCPS (UK), MSc Oral Biology (UK)
Department of Biomedical Dental Sciences
College of Dentistry
Imam Abdulrahman Bin Faisal University
Dammam, Saudi Arabia

Paul Anderson

BSc, PhD, MInstP CPhys
Dental Physical Science Unit
Institute of Dentistry
Queen Mary University of London
London, United Kingdom

WILEY Blackwell

This edition first published 2021
© 2021 John Wiley & Sons Ltd

All rights reserved. No part of this publication may be reproduced, stored in a retrieval system, or transmitted, in any form or by any means, electronic, mechanical, photocopying, recording or otherwise, except as permitted by law. Advice on how to obtain permission to reuse material from this title is available at http://www.wiley.com/go/permissions.

The right of Imran Farooq, Saqib Ali, and Paul Anderson to be identified as the authors of the editorial material in this work has been asserted in accordance with law.

Registered Offices
John Wiley & Sons, Inc., 111 River Street, Hoboken, NJ 07030, USA
John Wiley & Sons Ltd, The Atrium, Southern Gate, Chichester, West Sussex, PO19 8SQ, UK

Editorial Office
9600 Garsington Road, Oxford, OX4 2DQ, UK

For details of our global editorial offices, customer services, and more information about Wiley products visit us at www.wiley.com.

Wiley also publishes its books in a variety of electronic formats and by print-on-demand. Some content that appears in standard print versions of this book may not be available in other formats.

Limit of Liability/Disclaimer of Warranty
The contents of this work are intended to further general scientific research, understanding, and discussion only and are not intended and should not be relied upon as recommending or promoting scientific method, diagnosis, or treatment by physicians for any particular patient. In view of ongoing research, equipment modifications, changes in governmental regulations, and the constant flow of information relating to the use of medicines, equipment, and devices, the reader is urged to review and evaluate the information provided in the package insert or instructions for each medicine, equipment, or device for, among other things, any changes in the instructions or indication of usage and for added warnings and precautions. While the publisher and authors have used their best efforts in preparing this work, they make no representations or warranties with respect to the accuracy or completeness of the contents of this work and specifically disclaim all warranties, including without limitation any implied warranties of merchantability or fitness for a particular purpose. No warranty may be created or extended by sales representatives, written sales materials or promotional statements for this work. The fact that an organization, website, or product is referred to in this work as a citation and/or potential source of further information does not mean that the publisher and authors endorse the information or services the organization, website, or product may provide or recommendations it may make. This work is sold with the understanding that the publisher is not engaged in rendering professional services. The advice and strategies contained herein may not be suitable for your situation. You should consult with a specialist where appropriate. Further, readers should be aware that websites listed in this work may have changed or disappeared between when this work was written and when it is read. Neither the publisher nor authors shall be liable for any loss of profit or any other commercial damages, including but not limited to special, incidental, consequential, or other damages.

Library of Congress Cataloging-in-Publication Data

Names: Farooq, Imran, 1984– editor. | Ali, Saqib, 1985– editor. | Anderson,
    Paul (Professor of oral biology), 1959– editor.
Title: An illustrated guide to oral histology / edited by Imran Farooq,
    Saqib Ali, Paul Anderson.
Description: First edition. | Hoboken, NJ : Wiley, 2021. | Includes
    bibliographical references and index.
Identifiers: LCCN 2020038283 (print) | LCCN 2020038284 (ebook) | ISBN
    9781119669449 (cloth) | ISBN 9781119669548 (adobe pdf) | ISBN
    9781119669609 (epub)
Subjects: MESH: Mouth–anatomy & histology | Atlas
Classification: LCC QP146 (print) | LCC QP146 (ebook) | NLM WU 17 | DDC
    612.3/1–dc23
LC record available at https://lccn.loc.gov/2020038283
LC ebook record available at https://lccn.loc.gov/2020038284

Cover Design: Wiley
Cover Images: Imran Farooq

Set in 9.5/12.5pt STIXTwoText by SPi Global, Pondicherry, India
Printed and bound in Singapore by Markono Print Media Pte Ltd

10 9 8 7 6 5 4 3 2 1

Contents

Preface

It gives us great pleasure to present our book that addresses problems with respect to the teaching and learning of oral histology. The idea to write a book focused on important details of oral histological features popped up around two years ago, when we felt there are many deficient areas in the present literature concerning the said topic. This book gives information about these features in a user-friendly format. It contains high-definition (HD) histological images of oral tissues with integrated text containing their introduction, key identifying histological features, and clinical significance. The textbook is intended for dental undergraduate and postgraduate students, license examination aspirants, and oral histology instructors. We strongly believe that the book will suit the needs of professionals in each of these disciplines.

We would like to mention here that we do not wish the present book to be a substitution of more general textbooks in oral histology. It is our belief that a good dental practitioner not only needs strong clinical skills, but also a solid understanding of basic sciences. Consequently, our book should be considered as providing the first step of the ladder in learning oral histology. This book is aimed at encouraging students to pursue a more exhaustive appreciation of the subject. To counter technology needs and in-line with the digital age, a companion website for the book has also been developed.

Finally, we do not imagine ourselves to be error-free, and would always be open to criticism. Your suggestions to improve the book are greatly appreciated.

Imran Farooq
Saqib Ali
Paul Anderson

Sample Preparation

This atlas contains images obtained through hematoxylin and eosin (H and E) staining, micro-computed tomography (micro-CT), ground sectioning, and scanning electron microscopy (SEM). The steps for the preparation of samples and collection of images are as follows.

Hematoxylin and Eosin (H and E) Stained Sections

The tissues were stored in 10% buffered formalin prior to their use. The hard tissue samples were decalcified in 8% formic acid. The tissues (hard and soft) were washed with distilled water and then transferred into alcohol solution for the dehydration procedure. Post-dehydration, the samples were cleared in xylene solution. The tissues after clearing were shifted into soft paraffin and hard paraffin baths. The sections were blocked by embedding in hard paraffin and thin sections of 7 μm were taken from blocked tissues using microtome. H and E staining was performed, samples were dehydrated, and cover slips were placed using DPX mounting medium.

Micro-computed Tomography (Micro-CT)

The tissue blocks to observe enamel and dentin were prepared by cutting the roots with a high-speed handpiece. The anatomical crown portion was retained and a micro-CT machine (SkyScan 1172, version 1.5; Bruker Micro-CT, Kontich, Belgium) was used to obtain images of enamel and dentin. The images were obtained by scanning the samples using a voltage source of 100-KV, source current of 100-μA, pixel size of 27.45-μm, and exposure time of 1600 msec. In addition, 360° rotation, filter of Al + Cu and, Tagged Image File Format (TIFF) were used. The raw images were recreated using the NRecon software (Bruker SkyScan, Aartselaar, Belgium). The TIFF images were later converted to Joint Photographic Experts Group (JPEG) format using Microsoft Paint® software.

Ground Sections

For each ground section preparation, freshly extracted teeth were collected and fixed in acrylic blocks. The teeth were sectioned using a water-cooled diamond saw (Isomet® 5000 Linear Precision Saw, Buehler Ltd, IL, USA) longitudinally (for longitudinal sections) and horizontally (for transverse sections) to split the tooth into two parts. Each thick section of tooth was then grinded on carborundum stone with equal digital pressure to make the sections paper thin. The sections were then dehydrated in absolute alcohol for 10 minutes and clearing was then performed in xylene solution for 15 minutes. The section was mounted on to a glass slide using DPX mounting medium. Coverslip was then placed on top of the section carefully to avoid air entrapment.

Scanning Electron Microscopy

To observe dentinal tubules, SEM was performed. Dentin discs of 1.5 mm were first made by cutting the teeth horizontally over cemento-enamel junction using a precision saw (Isomet® 5000 Linear Precision Saw, Buehler Ltd, IL, USA). The discs were exposed to ethylenediaminetetraacetic acid (EDTA) for one minute to unblock the dentinal tubules. After washing them with distilled water for one minute and post air drying, these discs were mounted on stubs and sputter coated with gold. The discs were observed in an SEM (FEI, Inspect F50, The Netherlands) to obtain micrographs of dentinal tubules.

About the Editors

Dr. Imran Farooq
Dr. Imran Farooq graduated from Baqai Dental College, Karachi, Pakistan in 2007, and then worked in the same institute as a Clinical Demonstrator (Restorative Dentistry) for two years before joining Queen Mary, University of London (QMUL), UK, for his postgraduation in Oral Biology. After graduation from QMUL in 2011, he joined the College of Dentistry, Imam Abdulrahman Bin Faisal University, Dammam, Saudi Arabia, in 2012. He is currently working as an Assistant Professor in the Oral Biology Division. He has 10+ years' experience in teaching oral biology and histology to dental students. He has published 70+ research articles and book chapters that have received 700+ citations to date. His research interests include biomaterials, dental materials, hard tissue mineralization, and dental education.

Dr. Saqib Ali
Dr. Saqib Ali graduated from Baqai Dental College, Karachi, Pakistan in 2009, and then joined QMUL, UK, to pursue his postgraduation in Oral Biology. After graduating from QMUL in 2011, he worked as an Assistant Professor in the Oral Biology Department of Sardar Begum Dental College and Khyber College of Dentistry, Peshawar, Pakistan, and then, since 2016, he has been working as a faculty member (Course Director Oral Biology) in College of Dentistry, Imam Abdulrahman Bin Faisal University, Dammam, Saudi Arabia. He has 10+ years' experience in teaching oral biology and histology to dental students. He has published 40+ research articles and book chapters that have received 200+ citations to date. His research interests include biomaterials, dental materials, hard tissue mineralization, and dental education.

Prof. Paul Anderson
Prof. Paul Anderson graduated from Leeds in Biophysics and then completed a PhD in Biophysics in relation to Dentistry at the London Hospital Medical College (now part of QMUL). He has supervised 15 PhD students to completion, and has given invited research seminars in the Europe, the United States, Australia, New Zealand, Beijing, Hong Kong, and Malaysia. He is currently an associate editor of Caries Research, and Hon. Asst. Secretary of British Society for Oral and Dental Research (BSODR). He is also chair of the Institute of Dentistry Dental Postgraduate Committee. In 2011, he started the UK's first ever MSc in Oral Biology program in the United Kingdom, with now over 100 graduates. He has published 150+ research articles and book chapters that have received 2000+ citations to date. His research interests include X-ray microscopy, enamel and hydroxyapatite chemistry, and the biophysical chemical effects of salivary proteins in dental hard tissue protection.

List of Contributors

Amr Bugshan
Department of Biomedical Dental Sciences
College of Dentistry
Imam Abdulrahman Bin Faisal University
Dammam, Saudi Arabia

Saqlain Gilani
Department of Oral Biology
Islamic International Dental College
Riphah International University
Islamabad, Pakistan

Shehriar Husain
Department of Dental Materials Science
Sindh Institute of Oral Health Sciences
Jinnah Sindh Medical University
Karachi, Pakistan

Erum Khan
CODE-M Center of Dental Education &
Medicine
Karachi, Pakistan
and
Bhitai Dental and Medical College
Liaquat University of Medical and Health
Sciences,
Jamshoro, Pakistan

Syed Ali Khurram
Unit of Oral and Maxillofacial Pathology
School of Clinical Dentistry
University of Sheffield
Sheffield, United Kingdom

Zohaib Khurshid
Department of Prosthodontics and Dental
Implantology
College of Dentistry

King Faisal University
Al Ahsa, Saudi Arabia

Juzer Shabbir
Department of Operative Dentistry and
Endodontics
Liaquat College of Medicine and Dentistry
Karachi, Pakistan

Faraz Mohammed
Department of Biomedical Dental Sciences
College of Dentistry
Imam Abdulrahman Bin Faisal University
Dammam, Saudi Arabia

Fizza Saher
Department of Oral Biology
College of Dentistry
Ziauddin University
Karachi, Pakistan

Rizwan Ullah
Department of Oral Biology
Sindh Institute of Oral Health Sciences
Jinnah Sindh Medical University
Karachi, Pakistan

Muhammad Sohail Zafar
Department of Restorative Dentistry
College of Dentistry
Taibah University, Al Madinah
Al Munawwarah, Saudi Arabia
and
Department of Dental Materials
Islamic International Dental College
Riphah International University
Islamabad, Pakistan

About the Companion Website

This book is accompanied by a website at:

www.wiley.com/go/farooq/oral_histology

Scan the QR code:

The website includes:

- PowerPoint of figures
- Sample preparation

1

Tooth Development

Saqib Ali[1], Imran Farooq[1], and Syed Ali Khurram[2]

[1]*Department of Biomedical Dental Sciences, College of Dentistry, Imam Abdulrahman Bin Faisal University, Dammam, Saudi Arabia*
[2]*Unit of Oral and Maxillofacial Pathology, School of Clinical Dentistry, University of Sheffield, Sheffield, United Kingdom*

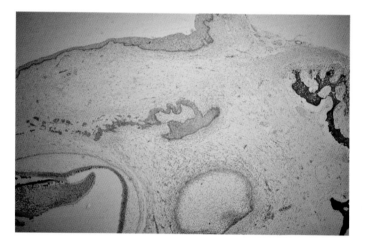

Figure 1.1   H and E stained section showing tooth development.

Tooth development starts on the 37th day of gestation with the formation of primary epithelial bands in the place of future upper and lower jaws. These horse-shoe-shaped bands correspond to the future dental arches. These epithelial bands then form two ingrowths called dental lamina (lingually positioned) and vestibular lamina (buccally positioned). These ingrowths extend into the mesenchyme which is surrounded by the neural crest cells. The vestibular lamina proliferates within the mesenchyme and leads to the formation of the vestibule (between the cheek and tooth-bearing portion of the jaw). The dental lamina gives rise to epithelial outgrowths toward the mesenchyme due to continuous proliferative activity which correspond to the location of forthcoming deciduous teeth. The tooth development is divided into the following stages: bud, cap, and bell (early and late). These stages along with the changes happening in the tooth germ are discussed in detail in the following sections.

An Illustrated Guide to Oral Histology, First Edition. Edited by Imran Farooq, Saqib Ali, and Paul Anderson.
© 2021 John Wiley & Sons Ltd. Published 2021 by John Wiley & Sons Ltd.
Companion website: www.wiley.com/go/farooq/oral_histology

1.1 Bud Stage

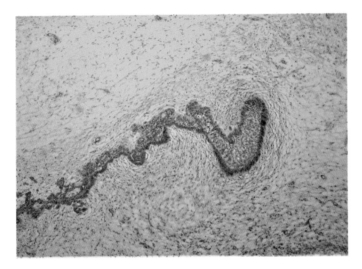

Figure 1.2 H and E stained section showing the bud stage of tooth development.

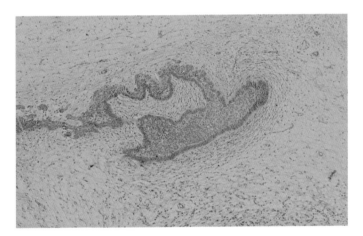

Figure 1.3 H and E stained section showing the bud stage of tooth development.

1.1.1 Description

The bud stage is the first stage of tooth development. It represents the first epithelial intrusion into the ectomesenchyme. The cells of the epithelium show minimal changes and the ectomesenchymal cells surround the epithelial bud. Due to the ectomesenchymal condensation (a process in which the epithelial bud propagates into the ectomesenchyme), the density of the cells increases near the epithelial outgrowth. This condensation is owed to the increased mitotic activity carried in the cells of the tooth bud and mesenchymal cells surrounding it. These buds develop at the distal side of the dental lamina and each bud represents a group of cells at dental lamina's end. The epithelial part is separated from the mesenchyme by a basement membrane. The ectomesenchyme surrounding the tooth bud is called the dental *follicle or sac* whereas the area directly subjacent to the condensation is called the *dental papilla*. The dental follicle is ultimately responsible for the formation of cementum, periodontal ligament (PDL), and alveolar bone. The dental papilla is responsible for the formation of dental pulp and dentin.

1.1.2 Key Identifying Features

The enamel organ at this stage appears roughly ovoid to spherical with poor histodifferentiation and morphodifferentiation. A typical tooth bud consists of centrally located polygonal (multiple-shaped) cells and peripherally arranged columnar cells.

1.1.3 Clinical Significance

The successful development of the tooth depends on the interaction of epithelial and mesenchymal components. If these parts grow individually, neither will differentiate further [1]. This epithelial–mesenchymal interaction starts in the bud stage; therefore, any problem affecting the bud stage could seriously affect the development of teeth.

1.2 Cap Stage

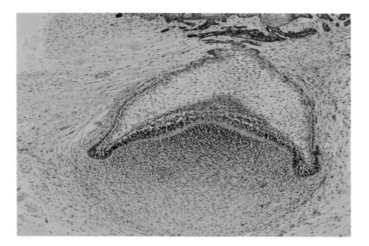

Figure 1.4   H and E stained section showing the cap stage of tooth development.

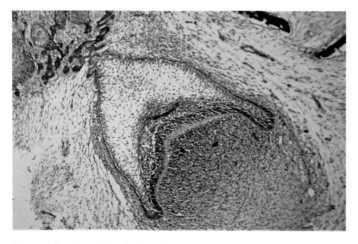

Figure 1.5   H and E stained section showing the cap stage of tooth development.

1.2.1 Description

The cap stage is the second stage of tooth development. As the tooth bud matures, it takes part of dental lamina along with it, which is called the lateral lamina. The tooth bud grows non-uniformly, and the growth is more in certain areas and less in others. This stage is called the cap stage as the epithelial outgrowth looks like a cap which is sitting on top of the condensed ectomesenchyme (dental papilla). During this stage, greater differentiation is seen in the central and peripheral cells. The central polygonal cells change into the stellate reticulum cells which have a somewhat star-shaped appearance due to greater intake of water, pushing the cells apart but retaining their desmosomal attachments. The peripheral cells change into external and inner enamel epithelium. The outer enamel epithelium cells are cuboidal whereas the inner epithelial cells are tall and columnar. These layers of epithelial cells are separated from the dental follicle and dental papilla by a basement membrane. Another structure called the *enamel knot* is formed during this stage which represents a collection of cells in the center of the inner enamel epithelium. It is a transitory structure which is believed to contribute cells to the *enamel cord (strand of cells)*.

1.2.2 Key Identifying Features

The enamel organ resembles a cap present on top of the dental papilla. The dental follicle and dental papilla become more recognizable during this stage compared to the bud stage.

1.2.3 Clinical Significance

It is believed that the blood supply of the tooth is established during the cap stage. The blood vessels first enter through the dental follicle, then move into the dental papilla [2]. Any disruptions during this stage could severely affect the vascular supply of the tooth and in turn, its maturation, vitality, and eruption.

1.3 Early Bell Stage

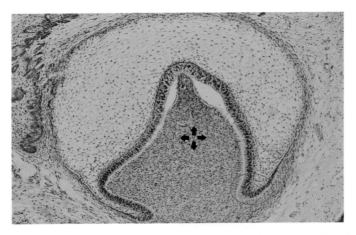

Figure 1.6 H and E stained section showing the early bell stage of tooth development (green circle, cervical loop; arrows, dental papilla).

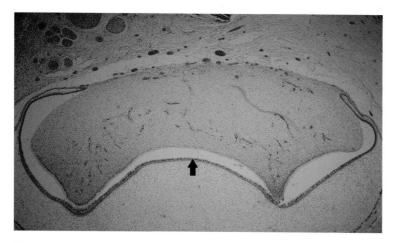

Figure 1.7 H and E stained section showing the early bell stage of tooth development (arrow, dental follicle).

1.3.1 Description

During this stage, the enamel organ resembles a bell. It is during this stage that the tooth crown will undertake its final shape (morphodifferentiation) and ameloblasts along with odontoblasts are histodifferentiated. The region where the outer and inner enamel epithelial cells meet at the border of enamel organ is called the *cervical loop*. In between the stellate reticulum and the inner enamel epithelial cells, some of the cell population differentiates and forms a new layer of cells called *stratum intermedium*. The cells of the inner enamel epithelium and stratum intermedium work collaboratively to form the enamel tissue. The enamel organ during the early bell stage clearly shows its four diverse layers: outer enamel epithelium, inner enamel epithelium, stellate reticulum, and stratum intermedium. During this stage, the enamel organ loses its contact with the oral epithelium as the dental lamina is broken down. This connection is restored during the process of tooth eruption. The remnants of dental lamina are called epithelial rest of Serres. In the early bell stage, the enamel knot disappears and the enamel cord appears between the stratum intermedium and stellate reticulum.

1.3.2 Key Identifying Features

On histological sections, bell-shaped enamel organ dissociated from the oral epithelium can be seen clearly. The tooth germ during this stage is enclosed by dental follicle. The cervical loop is also very prominent and easily recognizable.

1.3.3 Clinical Significance

Many important structures appear during this stage. It is believed that enamel cord facilitates the change from the cap to bell stage [1]. The cervical loop is responsible for the formation of Hertwig's epithelial root sheath (HERS) [3].

1.4 Late Bell Stage

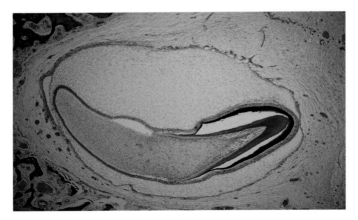

Figure 1.8 H and E stained decalcified section showing the late bell stage of tooth development.

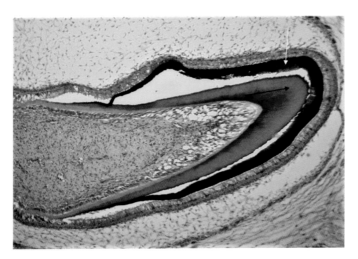

Figure 1.9 H and E stained decalcified section showing the late bell stage of tooth development (white arrow, enamel; black arrow, dentin).

1.4.1 Description

In the late bell stage, the tooth germ increases in size, and the hard tissues of the teeth start forming. The process of dentin formation is called *dentinogenesis* and it always precedes the process of enamel formation, i.e. *amelogenesis*. It is beyond the scope of this book to go into details of these processes but briefly, under the influence of inner enamel epithelium (which changes into pre-ameloblasts), the adjacent peripheral cells of dental papilla become odontoblasts. These odontoblasts start secreting of pre-dentin followed by dentin; this secretion stimulates pre-ameloblasts to change into ameloblasts which start secreting the enamel matrix (which mineralizes and becomes dental enamel later). While secreting, odontoblasts move away from the secretion area, leaving behind their odontoblastic processes. Similarly, ameloblasts migrate away from dentin while secreting enamel matrix. It should be noted that the formation of these two tissues begins in the area of future cusps/incisal edges and then slopes downward. This is the stage where the commencement of root formation begins as well.

1.4.2 Key Identifying Features

On the histological sections, prominently visible dental hard tissues (enamel and dentin) can be seen. Ameloblasts (on top of the newly formed enamel) and odontoblasts (just below the newly formed dentin) are also evident.

1.4.3 Clinical Significance

The visible development of HERS begins during this stage. The HERS is responsible for determining the shape, size, and number of roots [4]. Disruption to this stage could affect amelogenesis and dentinogenesis, leading to the formation of abnormal enamel and dentin, respectively (or non-formation) [5].

1.5 Root Formation

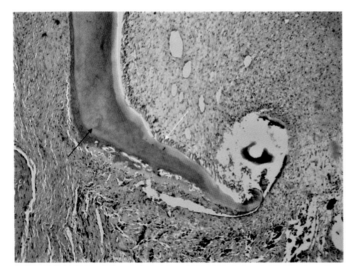

Figure 1.10 H and E stained section showing a tooth's root formation (white arrow, odontoblasts; black arrow, dentin).

1.5.1 Description

The tooth root has many important functions including anchorage of the tooth in maxilla/mandible and facilitating provision of blood supply (through apical foramina). The inside of the root is composed of radicular dentin and pulp canals whereas, on the outside, it is covered by a thin calcified layer of cementum. Root formation occurs because of the interaction between HERS, dental papilla, and dental follicle. After crown formation, the cervical loop grows apically as HERS circling dental papilla. The ectomesenchymal cells of dental papilla near the HERS change into odontoblasts and start secreting radicular dentin. The root dentin comes in contact with the dental follicle due to the perforation of HERS which leads to its mesh-network appearance. This contact changes dental follicular cells into cementoblasts (forming cementum), fibroblasts (forming PDL), and osteoblasts (forming alveolar bone). It should be noted that the HERS only maps the shape of the root and then disintegrates. Its remnants are known as epithelial cell rests of Malassez.

1.5.2 Key Identifying Features

On histological sections, developing root with prominent radicular dentin can be clearly seen just below a complete crown.

1.5.3 Clinical Significance

The HERS is responsible for determining the number of roots by forming a pair of tongue-shaped extensions that fuse [6]. Root formation plays an important role in tooth eruption. It is believed that with the pressure of the developing root, the crown of the tooth starts moving vertically to erupt in the oral cavity [7]. It should be noted, however, that there is evidence for rootless teeth to erupt [8] suggesting that it is a multifactorial process where root formation has a role, but it is not the only mechanism involved.

1.6 Amelogenesis Imperfecta (AI)

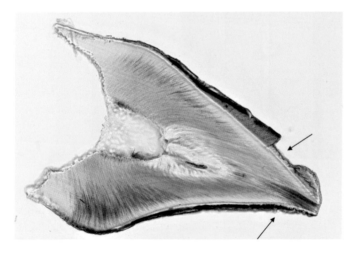

Figure 1.11 Low-power view of a ground section of a deciduous incisor showing irregular enamel surface (arrows) related to AI.

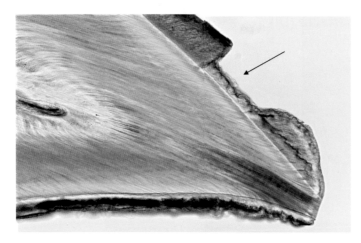

Figure 1.12 High-power view of a ground section of a deciduous incisor showing enamel pitting (arrow) related to AI.

1.6.1 Description

Amelogenesis imperfecta (AI) refers to a group of inherited genetic alterations that result in a defective enamel structure. AI is usually not associated with any syndrome or systemic disease. The teeth could appear yellow, brown, or sometimes grey. Several classifications have been suggested in the literature with the most commonly used one dividing AI into hypoplastic, hypomatured, and hypocalcified types. The hypoplastic type has insufficient amount of enamel matrix, the hypomature type has defective maturation of enamel whereas the hypocalcified type shows insufficient calcification of enamel. The genetic abnormalities in AI usually affect amelogenin (AMELX), enamelin (ENAM), kallikrein (KLK4), and matrix metalloproteinase 20 (MMP-20) genes. AI poses a significant clinical problem affecting the oral hygiene, masticatory function, and quality of life of the patient.

1.6.2 Key Identifying Features

On histological sections, it is difficult to identify the exact type of AI. However, reduced width/length of enamel along with pitting or clefts can be identified (ground sections) in addition to residual uncalcified enamel matrix (decalcified sections).

1.6.3 Clinical Considerations

Hypoplastic type is most common type of AI (60–73%) followed by hypomatured (20–40%) and hypocalcified (7%) types [9]. AI usually affects all the teeth of an individual and the diagnosis usually involves family history and clinical observation [10]. Radiographs reveal less than opaque enamel, especially when the mineralization has been affected [10]. The affected teeth are more prone to dental caries, dentinal sensitivity, and attrition [6]. Treatment options include masking of defective teeth with veneers and extra-coronal restorations [11].

1.7 Dentinogenesis Imperfecta (DI)

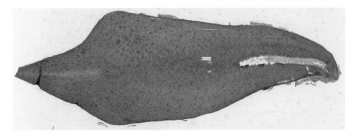

Figure 1.13 H and E stained decalcified section showing DI.

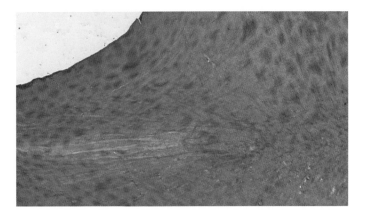

Figure 1.14 H and E stained decalcified section showing DI with a haphazard tubular architecture.

1.7.1 Description

Dentinogenesis imperfecta (DI) is a developmental hereditary condition (autosomal dominant) that affects the developing dentin. The dentin appears opalescent affecting both primary and permanent dentitions. DI can be classified into three main types: type I: DI associated with osteogenesis imperfecta; type II: DI similar to type I but not associated with osteogenesis imperfecta; and type III: initially reported in Brandywine population of Maryland and characterized by opalescent shell teeth (due to dentin hypotrophy) having marked attrition and large pulp chambers. As dentin forms the bulk of the tooth tissue, the teeth affected by DI are weak and prone to breakage and wear.

1.7.2 Key Identifying Features

On histological sections, teeth affected by DI show irregular dentinal tubules. In some areas, dentinal tubules can be completely absent. The dentin present can be quite irregular and haphazard and the pulp chamber can be quite small or completely obliterated.

1.7.3 Clinical Considerations

DI affects both dentitions and has an incidence of 1 in 6000 people [12]. The teeth have an amber color that ranges from yellow to brown or from blue to gray [13]. The normal scalloped interdigitation of dentin with enamel does not exist, and the flat enamel dentin junction leads to cracking of enamel followed by attrition of dentin [14]. The diagnosis is usually based on family history and the radiographical and clinical appearance of the teeth. Radiographically, the teeth usually have bulbous crowns with obliterated pulp chambers [12]. Clinically, the teeth are discolored with visible clinical defects and fractured enamel [5]. Treatment modalities include prosthetic crowns, over-dentures, orthodontic treatment (depending upon the severity), and dental implants (when all other conservative approaches have failed [12, 15]).

1.8 Dentin Dysplasia (DD)

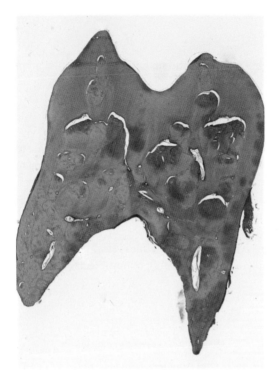

Figure 1.15 H and E stained decalcified section showing DD with haphazard coalescent globules of dentin and pulpal obliteration.

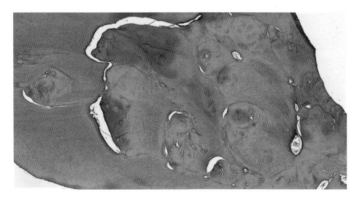

Figure 1.16 H and E stained decalcified section showing DD with the typical "water around the boulders" appearance.

1.8.1 Description

Dentin dysplasia (DD) is a rare genetic disorder that affects the development of dentin, mostly in radicular area. It can affect both dentitions, where the teeth have normal enamel but abnormal dentin with atypical pulp morphology. The first classification of DD was put forward by Witkop in the 1970s with DD divided into two types: DD-1 (radicular type) and DD-2 (coronal type) [16]. The teeth affected by DD-1 present with short, blunt roots with obliterated pulp chambers. In DD-2, teeth present with discoloration (brown to blue, amber colored, or opalescent), normal roots but enlarged pulp chambers (thistle tube appearance). The pulp chambers of primary teeth in DD-2 are almost completely obliterated whereas in permanent teeth, they may be partially obliterated.

1.8.2 Key Identifying Features

Histologically, irregular dentin with a disturbed tubular pattern, atubular areas, and globular atypical dentin masses inside pulp chambers can be seen.

1.8.3 Clinical Considerations

The etiology of this disease is still unclear. Wesley et al. previously proposed that it could be due to a problem with ameloblasts which leads to an abnormal differentiation of odontoblasts, leading to DD [17]. It was also proposed earlier that due to a problem with dental papilla (foci within it becoming calcified), DD develops as a result of less growth and/or obliteration of pulp chambers [18]. The diagnosis is based on clinical examination and radiographs. The teeth affected by DD have esthetic and functional abnormalities [19]. In addition, they are more prone to be mobile and are exfoliated prematurely [19]. The treatment options include stainless-steel crowns, endodontic therapy (although difficult due to obliteration of pulp chambers), removable dentures, and dental implants [20–22].

References

1 Berkovitz, B.K.B., Holland, G.R., and Moxham, B.J. (2009). *Oral Anatomy, Histology and Embryology*. Edinburgh: Mosby/Elsevier.
2 Nait Lechguer, A., Kuchler-Bopp, S., Hu, B. et al. (2008). Vascularization of engineered teeth. *J Dent Res* 87 (12): 1138–1143.
3 Luan, X., Ito, Y., and Diekwisch, T.G. (2006). Evolution and development of Hertwig's epithelial root sheath. *Dev Dyn* 235 (5): 1167–1180.
4 Li, J., Parada, C., and Chai, Y. (2017). Cellular and molecular mechanisms of tooth root development. *Development* 144 (3): 374–384.
5 Seow, W.K. (2014). Developmental defects of enamel and dentine: challenges for basic science research and clinical management. *Aust Dent J* 59 (Suppl 1): 143–154.
6 Kwon, H.-J.E. and Jiang, R. (1854). Development of the teeth. *Am J Dent Sci* 4 (2): 291–294.
7 Huang, X.F. and Chai, Y. (2012). Molecular regulatory mechanism of tooth root development. *Int J Oral Sci* 4 (4): 177–181.
8 Wang, X.P. (2013). Tooth eruption without roots. *J Dent Res* 92 (3): 212–214.
9 Chaudhary, M., Dixit, S., Singh, A., and Kunte, S. (2009). Amelogenesis imperfecta: report of a case and review of literature. *J Oral Maxillofac Pathol* 13 (2): 70–77.

10 Crawford, P.J., Aldred, M., and Bloch-Zupan, A. (2007). Amelogenesis imperfecta. *Orphanet J Rare Dis* 2: 17.

11 Chen, C.F., Hu, J.C., Bresciani, E. et al. (2013). Treatment considerations for patient with amelogenesis imperfecta: a review. *Braz Dent Sci* 16 (4): 7–18.

12 Barron, M.J., McDonnell, S.T., Mackie, I., and Dixon, M.J. (2008). Hereditary dentine disorders: dentinogenesis imperfecta and dentine dysplasia. *Orphanet J Rare Dis* 3: 31.

13 Gama, F.J.R., Corrêa, I.S., Valerio, C.S. et al. (2017). Dentinogenesis imperfecta type II: a case report with 17 years of follow-up. *Imaging Sci Dent* 47 (2): 129–133.

14 Sapir, S. and Shapira, J. (2001). Dentinogenesis imperfecta: an early treatment strategy. *Pediatr Dent* 23 (3): 232–237.

15 Subramaniam, P., Mathew, S., and Sugnani, S.N. (2008). Dentinogenesis imperfecta: a case report. *J Indian Soc Pedod Prev Dent* 26: 85–87.

16 Kim, J.W. and Simmer, J.P. (2007). Hereditary dentin defects. *J Dent Res* 86 (5): 392–399.

17 Wesley, R.K., Wysoki, G.P., Mintz, S.M., and Jackson, J. (1976). Dentin dysplasia type I. Clinical, morphologic, and genetic studies of a case. *Oral Surg Oral Med Oral Pathol* 41 (4): 516–524.

18 Logan, J., Becks, H., Silverman, S. Jr., and Pindborg, J.J. (1962). Dentin dysplasia. *Oral Surg* 15: 317.

19 Komlós, G., Joób-Fancsaly, Á., Pataky, L. et al. (2015). Difficulties in differential diagnosis of dentin dysplasia. Case report. *Fogorv Sz* 108 (2): 53–56.

20 Byahatti, S.M. (2013). Dentin dysplasia type I: a rare case report. *Int J Oral Health Sci* 3: 57–60.

21 Ravanshad, S. and Khayat, A. (2006). Endodontic therapy on a dentition exhibiting multiple periapical radiolucencies associated with dentinal dysplasia type 1. *Aust Endod J* 32 (1): 40–42.

22 Muñoz-Guerra, M.F., Naval-Gías, L., Escorial, V., and Sastre-Pérez, J. (2006). Dentin dysplasia type I treated with onlay bone grafting, sinus augmentation, and osseointegrated implants. *Implant Dent* 15 (3): 248–253.

2

Dental Enamel

Imran Farooq[1], Saqib Ali[1], and Paul Anderson[2]

[1] Department of Biomedical Dental Sciences, College of Dentistry, Imam Abdulrahman Bin Faisal University, Dammam, Saudi Arabia
[2] Dental Physical Science Unit, Institute of Dentistry, Queen Mary University of London, London, United Kingdom

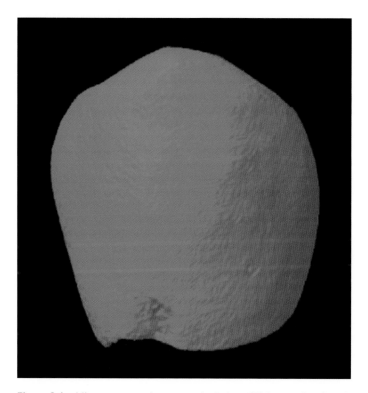

Figure 2.1 Micro-computed tomography (micro-CT) image showing dental enamel.

Dental enamel forms the protective covering of the crown of a tooth. It is formed of a hard calcified layer, present on all the clinically visible tooth surfaces in the oral cavity. Enamel by volume is composed of 96% inorganic material and 4% organic material and water. The inorganic material is composed of hydroxyapatite (HAP) crystals. This composition and its hierarchical

An Illustrated Guide to Oral Histology, First Edition. Edited by Imran Farooq, Saqib Ali, and Paul Anderson.
© 2021 John Wiley & Sons Ltd. Published 2021 by John Wiley & Sons Ltd.
Companion website: www.wiley.com/go/farooq/oral_histology

structure makes it the hardest structure of the human body; considerably harder than bone, dentin, and cementum. However, this composition should make enamel a highly brittle structure, but its structural arrangements and a layer of resistant underlying dentin helps it to maintain its structural integrity. Enamel is thickest over the cusps (~2.5 mm) and thinnest at the cervical margin of a tooth. The enamel-forming cells are called ameloblasts, but these cells are lost due to apoptosis and regression, once they complete their function. Therefore, enamel once formed, does not have the ability to use these cells for regeneration or repair. The hardness of enamel varies at different regions; surface enamel is harder and less porous than subsurface enamel. One reason for this is the ionic substitutions that take place between the surface enamel and saliva. Although considered a mineralized cell-less tissue (no ability to regenerate), enamel still permits ionic exchange with the ions of saliva. Another ion not derived from saliva which is incorporated into the enamel structure is fluoride, which can replace some of the hydroxyl ions in the HAP crystal lattice structure converting it to fluorapatite (FAP) which is more chemically stable and resistant to acidic attack. Other ions that can be substituted inside the enamel lattice structure and their resultant impact on the properties of the crystal lattice are summarized in Table 2.1.

Table 2.1 The impact of the replacement of enamel hydroxyapatite groups/ions with external ions on the crystal lattice.

External ion	Ion replaced in the crystal lattice	Overall impact
Carbonate	Phosphate or hydroxyl	Destabilizing effect
Magnesium	Calcium	Destabilizing effect
Fluoride	Hydroxyl	Stabilizing effect

Enamel's structure is complex and its physical properties vary at different regions but overall, it retains high impact/shearing strength but low tensile strength. The physical properties of enamel are summarized in Table 2.2.

Table 2.2 Important physical properties of enamel.

Physical property	Enamel
Knoop hardness number	296
Compressive strength	$76 \, MN/m^2$
Tensile strength	$46 \, MN/m^2$

MN = meganewtons ($N \times 10^6$).
Source: From ref. [1]. © 2009 Reprinted with permission of Elsevier.

2.1   Surface Enamel and Ionic Substitution

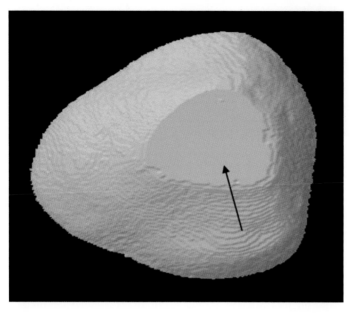

Figure 2.2   Micro-CT image showing surface enamel (arrow, ground and polished enamel).

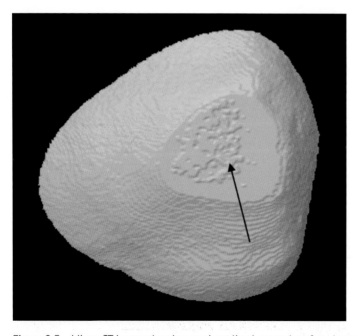

Figure 2.3   Micro-CT image showing remineralized enamel surface (arrow, ionic agglomerates formed due to ionic substitution on enamel's surface).

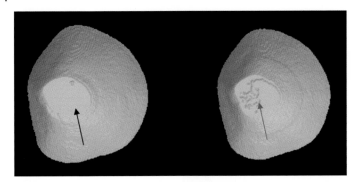

Figure 2.4 Micro-CT image showing enamel surface (black arrow, ground and polished surface; blue arrow, ionic agglomerates formed due to remineralization of enamel).

2.1.1 Description

The surface of enamel is in contact with the external environment. Salivary components are in constant contact with it. Ions originated from saliva and the external environment are responsible for changing the structure of the enamel surface through ionic substitution. Fluoride ions can replace hydroxyl ions in the apatite lattice structure and change HAP into FAP, which is more chemically stable. The process of losing enamel minerals after an acidic attack is called demineralization. Whereas, the restoration of these minerals back into the enamel surface is called remineralization. Figure 2.2 shows micro-CT image of an enamel surface which was ground and polished to give a flat surface. Figure 2.3 shows a remineralized enamel surface. Figure 2.4 shows two micro-CT images in which the precipitation of ions during remineralization can be clearly seen after the enamel's surface was exposed to fluoride solution after 24 hours. Precipitation of ions occurs due to the fact that the presence of fluoride enhances precipitation of calcium and phosphate ions on the surface.

2.1.2 Key Identifying Features

The surface enamel shows ionic agglomerates upon remineralization which can be detected when the surface is examined with certain techniques like micro-CT.

2.1.3 Clinical Significance

The oral cavity experiences cycles of demineralization and remineralization every day [2]. As enamel is a tissue which has no cellular regeneration competence, ionic substitution makes the surface structure harder and more resistant to acidic attack [3]. The conversion of HAP into FAP due to incorporation of fluoride ions into the HAP lattice structure makes the resultant enamel mineral less soluble and thus more cariostatic. Dental caries is a disease in which demineralization is the major step [4]. The benefit of fluoride on enamel's surface has encouraged its use in dentistry including its incorporation into mouthwashes, dentifrices, varnishes, and gels has increased over the last two decades [4].

2.2   Enamel Striae

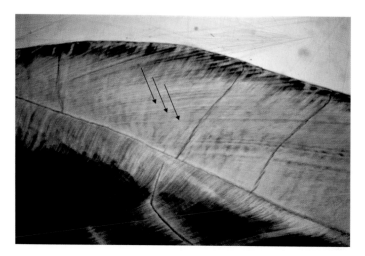

Figure 2.5   Ground section of enamel and dentin (arrows, enamel striae).

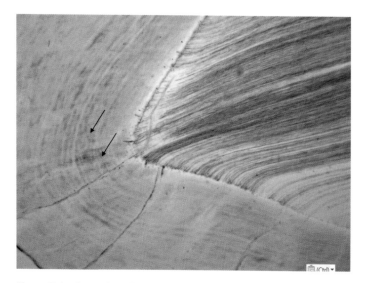

Figure 2.6   Ground section of enamel and dentin (arrows, enamel striae).

2.2.1   Description

Enamel striae or striae of retzius are incremental lines of enamel formed during the process of amelogenesis. The striae appear during the so-called rest period throughout amelogenesis in which ameloblastic activity is slowed down at consistent intervals. These lines represent the disparity in the calcification rhythms of the enamel matrix during formation. They are present throughout enamel as lines that are oblique to the enamel prism direction, and extend from the enamel dentin

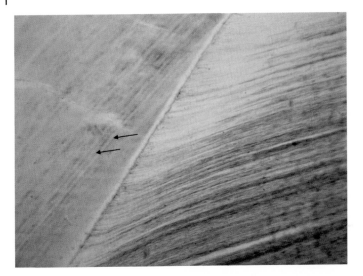

Figure 2.7 Ground section of enamel and dentin (arrows, enamel striae).

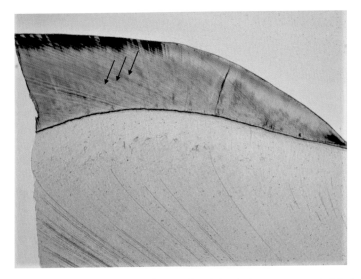

Figure 2.8 Ground section of enamel and dentin (arrows, enamel striae).

junction (EDJ) to the outer surface. Unlike other calcified tissues, enamel does not have the ability for cellular remodeling or repair, and therefore the striae remain intact after their initial formation. These striae are usually 25–30 μm apart and contain 7–10 cross striations (daily incremental lines) between them. At the outer surface they run in grooves called perikymata which are separated by ridges called perikymata ridges.

2.2.2 Key Identifying Features

In ground sections observed in a light microscope (Figures 2.5–2.8), striae can be seen as brown bands on the enamel surface. They are more prominent in postnatal enamel than prenatal enamel, they appear as oblique lines on longitudinal ground sections, and as concentric rings on transverse ground sections (resembling annual aging rings of a tree).

2.2.3 Clinical Significance

Striae are normal developmental features and show difference in rhythm as the tooth enamel matrix mineralizes [5]. The inter-striae distance can be used to estimate the time taken for crown formation and thus help in age identification in forensic odontology [1]. All parts of enamel develop at the same time in any individual, and will have the same pattern of formation and thus it can be called a fingerprint of enamel formation for a specific individual [6]. Some researchers believe that striae can be useful in predicting enamel growth trajectories [7].

2.3 Enamel Lamellae

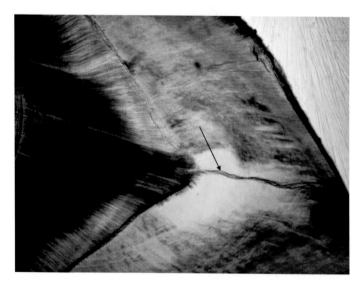

Figure 2.9 Ground section of enamel and dentin (arrow, enamel lamellae).

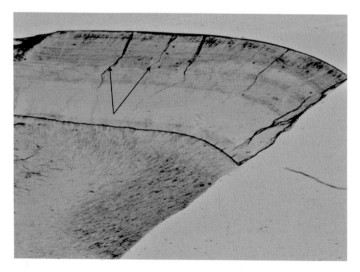

Figure 2.10 Ground section of enamel and dentin (arrows, enamel lamellae).

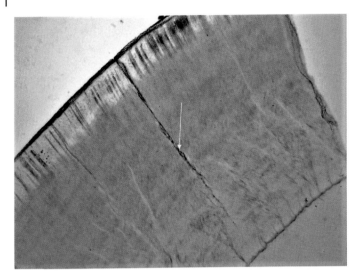

Figure 2.11 Ground section of enamel and dentin (arrow, enamel lamellae).

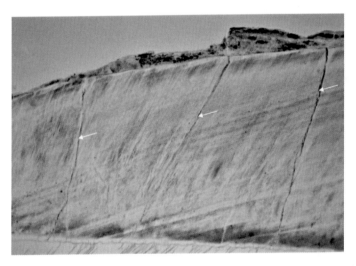

Figure 2.12 Ground section of enamel and dentin (arrows, enamel lamellae).

2.3.1 Description

Enamel lamellae are linear mineralization defects present in the enamel of both deciduous and permanent teeth. These are hypomineralized features of enamel and can extend various depths into enamel. These are structural faults that run through the entire thickness of enamel, and sometimes can cross the EDJ and enter dentin as well. They are sometimes observable on longitudinal ground sections, but are best seen in transverse ground sections. Their appearance is thought to be due to incomplete maturation of groups of prisms. Enamel lamellae can also contain degenerated cells, organic debris, and hypocalcified rod segments. Lamellae present on the proximal surface can be detected by transillumination but those present under occlusal fissures require sectioning of teeth to be observed.

2.3.2 Key Identifying Features

Enamel lamellae appear as large cracks, and can have varying depths, but are actually different from true cracks. Decalcification of a ground section can help to differentiate between a true crack and enamel lamellae. A true crack upon decalcification disappears while lamellae will persist.

2.3.3 Clinical Significance

Bodecker, 1906, was the first to describe enamel lamellae as developmental defects [8]. Gottlieb studied these defects extensively and proposed that they are caused by the hypocalcification of teeth [9]. It has been suggested that these lamellae are sites of weakness in a tooth and could act as an entry portal for bacteria, leading to dentinal caries [10]. Hardwick and Manly conducted a study in which they reported a caries-free premolar tooth that displayed lamellae with a related dentinal lesion [11]. Walker et al. reported that lamellae are permeable channels through which bacteria (e.g. streptococcus mutans and/or lactobacilli) can gain access inside the tooth structure progressing the development of dental caries [12].

2.4 Enamel Spindles

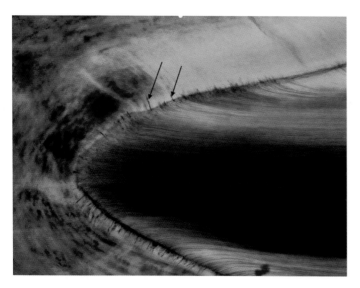

Figure 2.13 Ground section of enamel and dentin (arrows, enamel spindles).

2.4.1 Description

Enamel spindles form before enamel formation begins, with odontoblast processes that cross into dentin, enter the enamel and then get trapped within the ameloblast layer after amelogenesis starts, and are therefore entrapped extensions of odontoblasts. These club-shaped spindles are linear defects that have a different orientation to prisms and can extend up to many micrometers in enamel (~25 μm). Most spindles are found beneath the enamel cusps that occur at sites where most of the crowding of odontoblasts occurs. During the preparation of ground sections,

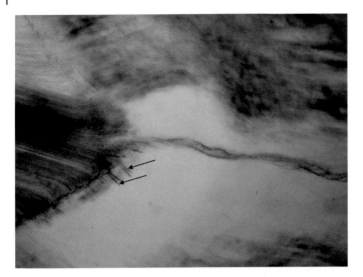

Figure 2.14 Ground section of enamel and dentin (arrows, enamel spindles).

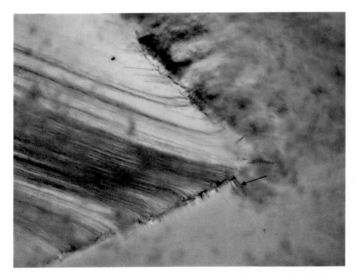

Figure 2.15 Ground section of enamel and dentin (arrow, enamel spindles).

drying can cause enamel spindles to lose their organic content and become trapped with air. These air-filled spindles can then appear black when viewed using an optical microscope under transmitted light. There are two reasons for the appearance of these spindles: (i) due to the extension of dentinal tubules which cross the EDJ and (ii) because of problems occurring during the amelogenesis process.

2.4.2 Key Identifying Features

Enamel spindles are extended continuations of dentinal tubules. Due to their orientation, they are best seen in longitudinal ground sections of enamel. They appear as short linear lines extending from the EDJ into enamel.

2.4.3 Clinical Significance

A previous transmission electron microscopy (TEM) study revealed that enamel spindles are continuous with dentinal tubules in human enamel and branch rarely [13]. Enamel spindles are hypomineralized structures which contain less calcium and phosphorous, as compared with enamel prisms [14]. Being the extensions of odontoblastic process, they can serve as pain receptors which explain the enamel hypersensitivity experienced by some patients during cavity preparations [15].

2.5 Enamel Tufts

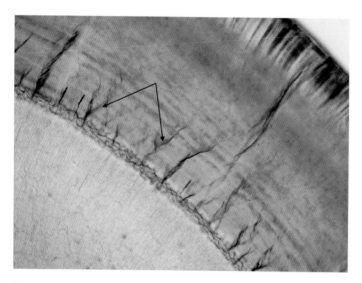

Figure 2.16 Ground section of enamel and dentin (arrows, enamel tufts).

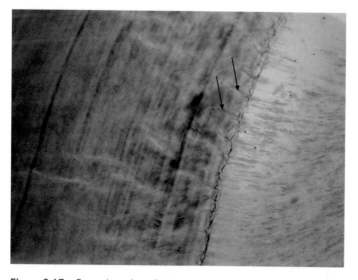

Figure 2.17 Ground section of enamel and dentin (arrows, enamel tufts).

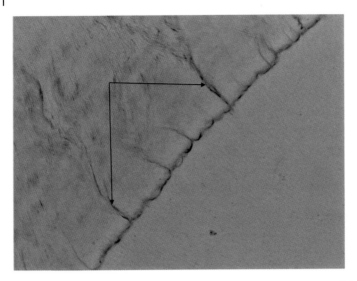

Figure 2.18 Ground section of enamel and dentin (arrows, enamel tufts).

2.5.1 Description

Enamel tufts are hypomineralized structures that project from the EDJ and usually continue in the enamel tissue for some distance. It is not clear if the hypomineralization is the same in all areas of enamel tufts. They contain increased quantities of protein as compared with the rest of the enamel. Tufts appear developmentally as mineralization faults or defects. They are present on the inner third of enamel and run parallel with the enamel prisms. One reason for their appearance is a sudden change in the direction of enamel rods arising from different areas of EDJ during developmental stages. Therefore, it has been suggested that these tufts contain hypocalcified enamel rods and inter-rod substances. They are hypomineralized assemblies which are not linked with dentinal tubules and are a cause of space creation in enamel.

2.5.2 Key Identifying Features

Enamel tufts are rarely seen on longitudinal ground sections and are best seen in transverse sections due to their arrangement and orientation. They are ribbon-like structures that appear as tufts of grass and are always branched. Similar to a tree, they have a stalk/trunk and twigs or branches. The branches are multiple and there is no specific number.

2.5.3 Clinical Significance

Enamel tufts may appear as a result of metabolic changes occurring in enamel during development [16]. Enamel tufts create spaces at the EDJ, and can provide a passageway for invading bacteria to dentinal tubules and, ultimately the dental pulp [17]. They are considered as one of the principal causes of fractures that develop in a tooth due to continuous overloading, but they are also stress-shielding entities due to their structural arrangements [18]. As enamel tufts are rich in proteins (13–17 kd sheath proteins) [19], propagation of cracks is slowed down further as the tufts are replenished by proteins [20].

2.6 Enamel Dentin Junction (EDJ)

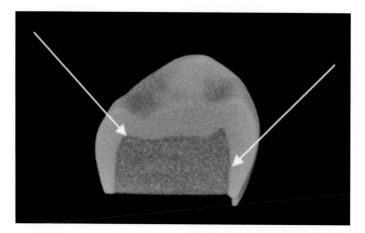

Figure 2.19 Micro-CT image of enamel and dentin (arrows, EDJ).

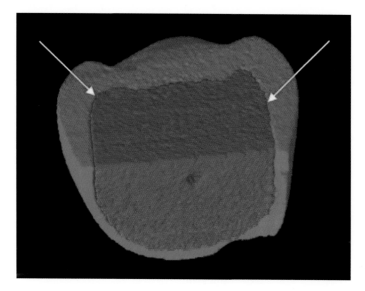

Figure 2.20 Micro-CT image of enamel and dentin (arrows, EDJ).

2.6.1 Description

The EDJ is formed between the enamel and dentin tissues. The EDJ forms a bond between these two distinct tissues; enamel being more brittle than the dentin. The EDJ is scalloped (not straight) and this structural feature provides a stronger connection between the two tissues. Scalloping at the EDJ is particularly common underneath cusps and incisal edges. Each indentation of the scallop represents the place where once ameloblasts resided. This junction is believed to be less mineralized than both the tissues. The development of the EDJ is marked by the presence of ameloblasts and a basement membrane in the bell stage of tooth formation. The EDJ is a complex structure where the three most important tooth tissues (cervical enamel, dentin, and cementum) are present, and it unites at least two dissimilar tissues (enamel and dentin).

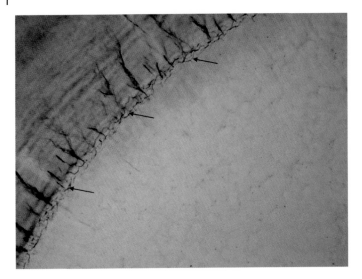

Figure 2.21 Ground section of enamel and dentin (arrows, EDJ).

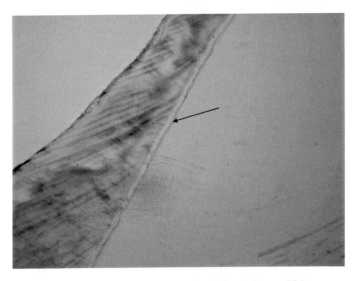

Figure 2.22 Ground section of enamel and dentin (arrow, EDJ).

2.6.2 Key Identifying Features

In the EDJ, scallops project from the enamel toward dentin. In ground sections, EDJ appears at the end of the brown-colored enamel tissue, and at the start of the black-colored dentin.

2.6.3 Clinical Significance

The EDJ acts as an anti-crack propagation area due to its lower mineralization, and its increased collagen content, both of which can disperse stresses [21]. Another function of the EDJ is to prevent delamination of the enamel from the dentin [22]. The von Korff fibers that extend from dentin into enamel also inhibit delamination [23]. The scallops of EDJ prevent the relative sliding of the two tissues, and increase its surface area, which ensures that the greatest number of fibers cross it to make the bond between the two tissues more stronger [23]. The exact mechanism of formation of these scallops is unknown, but it is anticipated that since enamel shrinks during maturation, this shrinking facilitates the formation of scallops [24].

2.7 Neonatal Line

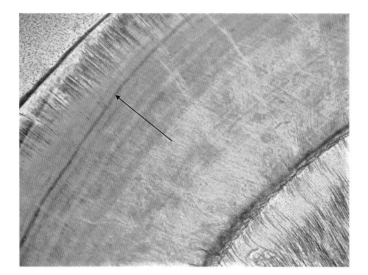

Figure 2.23 Ground section of enamel and dentin (arrow, neonatal line in enamel).

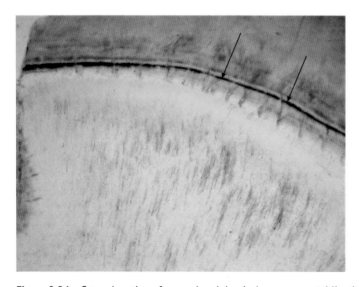

Figure 2.24 Ground section of enamel and dentin (arrow, neonatal line in enamel).

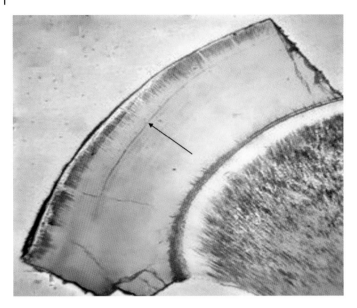

Figure 2.25 Ground section of enamel and dentin (arrow, neonatal line in enamel).

2.7.1 Description

The neonatal line is a marked single stria that appears at birth. It is a hypomineralized line resulting from significant metabolic changes that occur at birth. As the body is adapting to extra-uterine life, this leaves permanent marks in enamel. These changes are as biological landmarks, the appearance of the neonatal line is one. Since it is a prominent stria, it is considered as an exaggerated incremental line of enamel. It is believed that enamel prisms change their direction at the neonatal line. The enamel formed prior to birth is called prenatal enamel, and that formed after birth is called postnatal enamel. The neonatal line of enamel is only seen in teeth that are mineralizing at birth, i.e. all primary teeth and first permanent molar tooth. It is believed that prenatal enamel is better organized and developed than postnatal enamel, representing a well-protected and systematized environment during intrauterine (IU) life.

2.7.2 Key Identifying Features

The neonatal line appears dark brownish and can be visualized in both longitudinal and transverse ground sections. It is darker in color and larger than the other striae, and it follows the same direction of enamel striae in transverse sections. Therefore, it is sometimes also referred to as a "neonatal ring."

2.7.3 Clinical Significance

Enamel is the hardest tissue of the human body and therefore it resists postmortem changes [6]. The neonatal line has a great significance in forensic dentistry. The criminal act of neonaticide is still common in many countries and mostly involves the slaying of female babies [25]. The objective of an examination of skeletal remains (like tooth enamel) is to scrutinize claims of stillbirth and to separate these from infanticide [25]. It should be noted that most infanticides occur instantly after birth and a few days to a few weeks post-birth are required for postnatal enamel to fully develop and form the clear demarcation of a neonatal line [26]. It has been reported by Canturk et al. that prolonged stressful deliveries result in thicker neonatal lines, as opposed to an elective caesarean delivery, where the neonatal lines are thinner [27]. There is a linear relationship between the width of the neonatal line and the stress to which the infant was exposed during the course of birth.

2.8 Gnarled Enamel

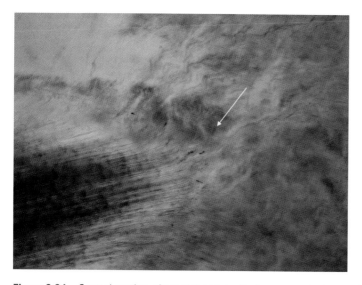

Figure 2.26   Ground section of enamel and dentin (arrow, gnarled enamel).

2.8.1 Description

Enamel rods or prims do not follow a straight course throughout their length. The spiral or twisted pattern of enamel prisms beneath cusps and incisal edges of teeth is called gnarled enamel. In gnarled enamel, prisms spiral over one another and appear more distinct and irregular. This arrangement of prisms from dentin toward the enamel surface is complex and complicated. Gnarled enamel is seen clearly on the ground sections under transmitted light near the EDJ and has an optical appearance. Gnarled enamel is more apparent when sections of teeth are cut in an oblique plane. The characteristic strength of gnarled enamel is not due to a difference in composition but rather only due to a spiral arrangement of enamel prisms.

2.8.2 Key Identifying Features

In gnarled enamel, the prisms are seen to interwine or spiral. The prisms of gnarled enamel appear disoriented; however, this disorientation gives this area its characteristic strength.

2.8.3 Clinical Significance

This gnarled appearance of enamel underneath cusps makes it resistant to fractures [28]. This zone of gnarled enamel is especially resistant to cleavage, unlike regular enamel [29]. Clinicians should be aware of the location of this area as it could be especially resistant to dental drill penetration during restorative procedures [30].

2.9 Enamel Caries

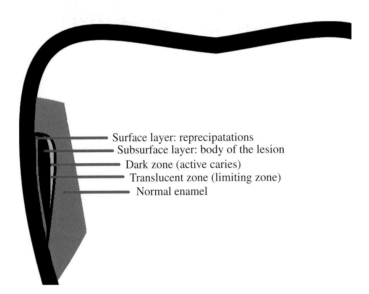

Surface layer: reprecipatations
Subsurface layer: body of the lesion
Dark zone (active caries)
Translucent zone (limiting zone)
Normal enamel

Figure 2.27 Diagrammatic representation of different zones of enamel caries.

2.9.1 Description

Dental enamel routinely goes through cycles of demineralization and remineralization in the oral environment. Under normal conditions, there is an equilibrium between these two processes. If this balance shifts toward demineralization, dental caries will ensue. Dental caries affecting only enamel (called enamel caries) has different zones as compared with the dentinal caries. The enamel caries is usually divided into four histological zones: the surface layer (where reprecipitations occur), the subsurface layer (also called as the body of the lesion), the dark zone (where carious lesion is progressing), and the translucent zone (which is a limiting zone). Enamel caries takes more time to progress compared to dentin.

2.9.2 Key Identifying Features

Enamel carious lesions are confined to the enamel tissues, and do not extend beyond EDJ.

2.9.3 Clinical Considerations

Dental caries confined to the enamel only have a specific treatment strategy. For enamel caries, nonoperative treatment protocol like the use of sealants and fluoride varnishes is recommended to arrest caries progression [31]. It should also be noted that non-cavitated carious lesions do not require restorative intervention. Noninvasive procedures are preferential for enamel-only lesions, and these lesions should be given a chance to remineralize naturally [32].

References

1 Berkovitz, B.K.B., Holland, G.R., and Moxham, B.J. (2009). *Oral Anatomy, Histology and Embryology*. Edinburgh: Mosby/Elsevier.

2 AlShehab, A.H., AlHazoom, A.A., Alowa, M.H. et al. (2018). Effect of bristle stiffness of manual toothbrushes on normal and demineralized human enamel: an in vitro profilometric study. *Int J Dent Hyg* 16 (2): e128–e132.

3 Farooq, I., Ali, S., Siddiqui, I.A. et al. (2019). Influence of thymoquinone exposure on the micro-hardness of dental enamel: an in vitro study. *Eur J Dent* 13 (3): 318–322.

4 Farooq, I., Majeed, A., AlShwaimi, E. et al. (2019). Efficacy of a novel fluoride containing bioactive glass based dentifrice in remineralizing artificially induced demineralization in human enamel. *Fluoride* 52 (3 Pt 3): 447–455.

5 Brand, R.W., Isselhard, D.E., and Elaine, S. (2003). *Anatomy of Orofacial Structures*, 269. St. Louis: Mosby. ISBN: 978-0-323-01954-5.

6 Chandrashekar, C., Takahashi, M., and Miyakawa, G. (2010). Enamel and forensic odontology: revealing the identity. *J Hard Tissue Biol* 19: 1–4.

7 Reid, D.J. and Ferrell, R.J. (2006). The relationship between number of striae of retzius and their periodicity in imbricational enamel formation. *J Hum Evol* 50 (2): 195–202.

8 Bodecker, C.F. (1906). Enamel of teeth decalcified by the celloidin method and examined with ultra-voilet light. *Dent Revy* 20: 317.

9 Gotlieb, B. (1944). The histopathy of dental caries. *J Dent Res* 23: 369–384.

10 Thoma, K. (1944). *Oral Pathology*, vol. 562. St. Louis: CV Mosby.

11 Hardwick, J.L. and Manly, E.B. (1952). Caries of the enamel. Part II. *Br Dent J* 92: 225–236.

12 Walker, B.N., Makinson, O.F., and Peters, M.C. (1998). Enamel cracks. The role of enamel lamellae in caries initiation. *Aust Dent J* 43 (2): 110–116.

13 Palamara, J., Phakey, P.P., Rachinger, W.A., and Orams, H.J. (1989). Ultrastructure of spindles and tufts in human dental enamel. *Adv Dent Res* 3 (2): 249–257.

14 Kumar, G.S. (2015). *Orban's Oral Histology & Embryology*, 14e. Elsevier.

15 Heymann, H.O., Swift, E.J., and Ritter, A.V. (2013). *Sturdevant's Art and Science of Operative Dentistry*. St. Louis: Elsevier/Mosby.

16 Beust, T.B. (1932). Occurrence of enamel tufts. *J Dent Res* 12: 601–608.

17 Bhaskar, S.N. and Orban, B.J. (1991). *Orban's Oral Histology and Embryology*. St. Louis: Mosby Year Book.

18 Chai, H., Lee, J.J., Constantino, P.J. et al. (2009). Remarkable resilience of teeth. *Proc Natl Acad Sci U S A* 106 (18): 7289–7293.

19 Amizuka, N., Uchida, T., Fukae, M. et al. (1992). Ultrastructural and immunocytochemical studies of enamel tufts in human permanent teeth. *Arch Histol Cytol* 55 (2): 179–190.

20 Roach, D.H., Lathabai, S., and Lawn, B.R. (1988). Interfacial layers in brittle cracks. *J Am Ceram Soc* 71: 97–105.

21 Shimizu, D. and Macho, G.A. (2007). Functional significance of the microstructural detail of the primate dentino-enamel junction: a possible example of exaptation. *J Hum Evol* 52 (1): 103–111.

22 Imbeni, V., Kruzic, J.J., Marshall, G.W. et al. (2005). The dentin-enamel junction and the fracture of human teeth. *Nat Mater* 4 (3): 229–232.

23 Lin, C.P., Douglas, W.H., and Erlandsen, S.L. (1993). Scanning electron microscopy of type I collagen at the dentin-enamel junction of human teeth. *J Histochem Cytochem* 41 (3): 381–388.

24 Starkey, W.E. (1971). Dimensional changes associated with enamel maturation in rabbits. *Arch Oral Biol* 16 (5): 479–493.

25 Janardhanan, M., Umadethan, B., Biniraj, K. et al. (2011). Neonatal line as a linear evidence of live birth: estimation of postnatal survival of a new born from primary tooth germs. *J Forensic Dent Sci* 3 (1): 8–13.

26 Whittaker, D.K. and MacDonald, D.G. (1989). *A Colour Atlas of Forensic Dentistry*, 1e, 58–66. England: Wolfe Publishing Ltd.

27 Canturk, N., Atsu, S.S., Aka, P.S., and Dagalp, R. (2014). Neonatal line on fetus and infant teeth: an indicator of live birth and mode of delivery. *Early Hum Dev* 90 (8): 393–397.

28 Nanci, A. and Ten, C.A.R. (2003). *Ten Cate's Oral Histology: Development, Structure, and Function.* St. Louis: Mosby.

29 Weber, D.F. (1973). Sheath configurations in human cuspal enamel. *J Morph* 141 (4): 479–489.

30 Fernandes, C.P. and Chevitarese, O. (1991). The orientation and direction of rods in dental enamel. *J Prosthet Dent* 65 (6): 793–800.

31 Fellows, J.L., Gordan, V.V., Gilbert, G.H. et al. (2014). Dentist and practice characteristics associated with restorative treatment of enamel caries in permanent teeth: multiple-regression modeling of observational clinical data from the National Dental PBRN. *Am J Dent* 27 (2): 91–99.

32 Rechmann, P., Doméjean, S., Rechmann, B.M. et al. (2016). Approximal and occlusal carious lesions: restorative treatment decisions by California dentists. *J Am Dent Assoc* 147 (5): 328–338.

3

Dentin

Imran Farooq[1], Saqib Ali[1], Syed Ali Khurram[2], and Paul Anderson[3]

[1] Department of Biomedical Dental Sciences, College of Dentistry, Imam Abdulrahman Bin Faisal University, Dammam, Saudi Arabia
[2] Unit of Oral and Maxillofacial Pathology, School of Clinical Dentistry, University of Sheffield, Sheffield, United Kingdom
[3] Dental Physical Science Unit, Institute of Dentistry, Queen Mary University of London, London, United Kingdom

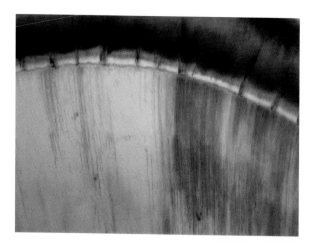

Figure 3.1 Ground section showing enamel (brown) and dentin (black and white).

Dentin is a calcified mineralized tissue like enamel but with a very different composition. It is the second hardest tissue in the human body after dental enamel, and contains by volume 70% inorganic material, 20% organic material, and 10% water. Dentin is produced by odontoblast cells that reside at the periphery of dental pulp. The cell bodies of these cells are present in the pulp whereas their processes, i.e. odonto-blastic processes, extend into the dentinal tubules. Dentinal tubules also contain fluid, and the movement of this fluid may be responsible for dentinal hypersensitivity (DH) which is characterized by a sharp pain of short duration. Dentin forms the bulk of tooth tissue and is present in both coronal and radicular portions of the teeth. The basic structural inorganic component of dentin is hydroxyapatite (HAP) crystals, but these crystals are very much smaller in size as compared to enamel. Dentin, unlike enamel, can be produced physiologically (secondary dentin) or in response to external stimuli (tertiary and scle-rotic dentin). A few important differences between enamel and dentin are summarized in Table 3.1.

Dentin is one of the major constituents of the tooth structure. The key components of dentin tissue are now discussed in detail in the following sections.

An Illustrated Guide to Oral Histology, First Edition. Edited by Imran Farooq, Saqib Ali, and Paul Anderson.
© 2021 John Wiley & Sons Ltd. Published 2021 by John Wiley & Sons Ltd.
Companion website: www.wiley.com/go/farooq/oral_histology

Table 3.1 Differences between enamel and dentin tissue.

	Enamel	Dentin
Embryological origin	Enamel organ	Dental papilla
Synthetic cells	Ameloblasts	Odontoblasts
Location	Covering the crown	Crown (covered by enamel) and root (covered by cementum)
Color	Translucent	Pale yellow
Mineral content	~96 wt.%	~70 wt.%
Crystal size	Bigger	Smaller
Hardness	More	Less
Brittleness	More	Less
Flexibility	Less	More
Compressive strength	Less	More
Tensile strength	Less	More
Flexural strength	Less	More
Surface energy	High	Low
Ability to regenerate	None	Yes

3.1 Dentinal Tubules

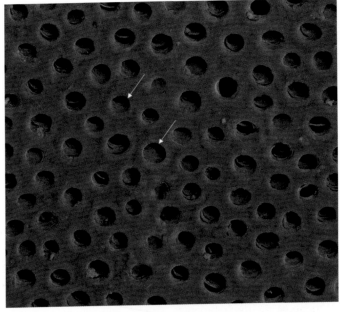

Figure 3.2 Scanning electron microscope (SEM) image of dentin (arrows, dentinal tubules).

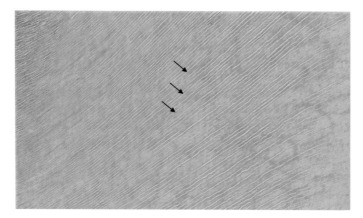

Figure 3.3 H and E stained decalcified section of dentin (arrows, dentinal tubules).

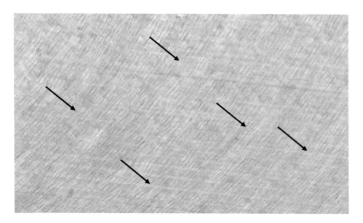

Figure 3.4 Ground section showing dentinal tubules (arrows).

3.1.1 Description

Dentinal tubules contain odontoblastic processes, dentinal fluid, and afferent nerve terminals. The odontoblastic processes are derived from the odontoblasts (dentin-forming cells). The odontoblasts are unique as they are present in two tissues at the same time, i.e. their cell body resides at the pulp periphery whereas the odontoblastic process is present inside dentinal tubules which are a part of dentin tissue. Dentinal tubules run from the EDJ toward the mineralization front and are present throughout dentin showing most abundant branching near the EDJ. Their thickness varies in different regions, being thicker near pulp and thinner near the EDJ. Their number also varies depending on the location with approximately 50 000–75 000 tubules/mm^2 seen near the pulpal surface. The dentin present between the tubules is called intertubular dentin whereas the dentin formed on the walls of tubules, narrowing its lumen is termed peritubular dentin.

3.1.2 Key Identifying Features

The dentinal tubules appear sigmoid (s-shaped) running between the pulp and the scalloped EDJ.

3.1.3 Clinical Significance

Movement of dentinal fluid upon exposure of these tubules clinically leads to DH [1]. The movement of fluid increases shear-stress on the nerve terminals of pulp causing dental pain [2]. DH is defined as sharp pain of short duration when a stimulus comes in contact with an exposed dentin surface [1], and this increasingly accepted hypothesized mechanism is known as the "hydrodynamic theory" [2]. The stimuli could be evaporative, tactile, osmotic, or chemical in origin. Management of DH includes occlusion of tubules by agents like fluoride or biomaterials such as bioactive glasses, desensitization of nerves by potassium salts, and use of dentin sealers [3].

3.2 Organic Matrix of Dentin

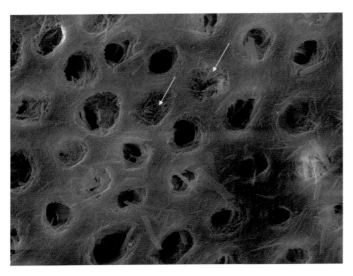

Figure 3.5 SEM image showing organic matrix of dentin covering dentinal tubules (arrows, mineralized collagen fibers).

3.2.1 Description

The organic matrix of dentin is mostly composed of collagen fibers which are protein in nature. A small proportion of it also comprises non-collagenous proteins which can act as promoters or inhibitors of mineralization. The collagen fibers in dentin have a high tensile strength and cover the superior surface of dentinal tubules. The collagen found in dentin is of type I mostly although traces of types III and V are also found. These collagen fibers come from the intertubular and peritubular dentin with the former being more dense and prominent compared to the latter, making peritubular dentin structure poor in collagen and much more mineralized than other parts of dentin. On the other hand, intertubular dentin contains a tightly interwoven network of type I collagen fibers. The formation of dentin is preceded by the development and deposition of an organic matrix first, the presence of which is supported by the presence of collagen fibers called von Korff fibers (which initially have type III collagen). With the growth of odontoblasts, type I collagen fibers take their place with an orientation parallel to the future EDJ.

3.2.2 Key Identifying Features

The organic matrix on the surface of dentin can be seen in the form of collagen fibers that appear as threads or string-like filaments covering spherical dentinal tubules which can be present both inside and outside the tubules.

3.2.3 Clinical Significance

The role of collagen fibers in dentin is like a scaffold that holds up minerals inside the holes/gaps of fibrils [4]. During the developmental stages, crystals in the form of calcospherites are deposited at various distant sites in the matrix and get trapped within the collagen [5]. This capture allows them to become stable in one place, thus helping in globular calcification of the dentin matrix [5]. As enamel, dentin is also deposited incrementally and changes in the collagen fiber orientation can be seen [5].

3.3 Primary and Secondary Curvatures of Tubules

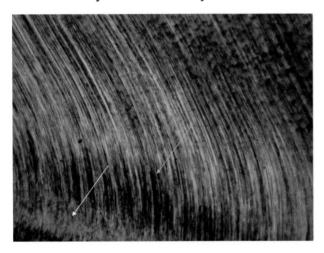

Figure 3.6 Ground section showing primary curvatures (orange arrow) and secondary curvatures (white arrow) of dentinal tubules.

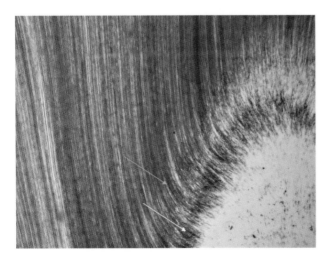

Figure 3.7 Ground section showing primary curvatures (orange arrow) and secondary curvatures (white arrow) of dentinal tubules.

3.3.1 Description

Primary dentin or circumpulpal dentin forms the bulk of the dentin structure. It is present in both coronoal and radicular dentin and is formed before root formation is complete. The outermost part of primary dentin near the EDJ is called mantle dentin which is slightly less mineralized. Secondary dentin which forms slowly throughout life is closer to the pulp. Its deposition is not uniform and with aging, continued deposition of secondary dentin could lead to narrowing, or reduction in the size of the pulp chamber. This phenomenon is called pulp recession. Both primary and secondary dentins have the same mineral to organic matrix ratio. Dentinal tubules follow a curved sigmoid course containing primary curvatures which are less pronounced in the root. In some areas, these tubules show a smaller change in direction called secondary curvatures. These curvatures are more prominent in the root area where the S-shaped curvatures smooth out taking a more linear course.

3.3.2 Key Identifying Features

The dentinal tubules possess sigmoid-shaped or s-shaped primary curvature. The secondary curvatures are more or less straight in direction. Dentinal tubules in primary dentin are more organized compared to secondary dentin.

3.3.3 Clinical Significance

In general, since dentin is less mineralized than enamel, the rate of caries spread is faster in dentin, especially along the direction of the dentinal tubules [6]. The formation of secondary dentin asymmetrically around the sides and roof of the pulp chamber could lead to a reduction in DH [7]. Iatrogenically, exposure of the pulp chamber in younger patients is more common than older patients as in the latter, pulp horns recede due to the deposition of secondary dentin on the roof of pulp chamber [5].

3.4 Interglobular Dentin

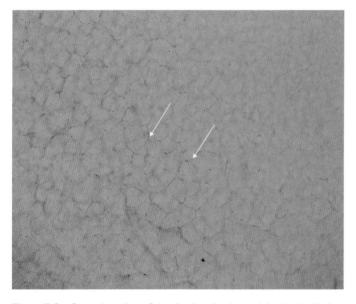

Figure 3.8 Ground section of dentin showing interglobular dentin (arrows).

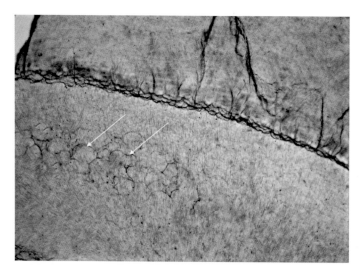

Figure 3.9 Ground section of dentin showing interglobular dentin (arrows).

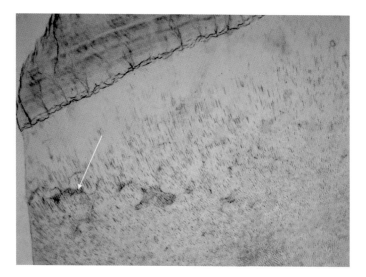

Figure 3.10 Ground section of dentin showing interglobular dentin (arrows).

3.4.1 Description

Interglobular dentin (IGD) could be defined as a hypomineralized or hypocalcified area in dentin. The mineralization of IGD could range from none to being slightly mineralized. The reason for its appearance is believed to be the non-fusion of calcospherites in this area to form a homogenous mass. A decrease in vitamin D or an increase of fluoride could be attributed as potential risk factors for IGD development. IGD is seen in circumpulpal dentin and dentinal tubules pass through these areas without any discontinuity. The probable reason for this could be the fact that IGD is a result of reduced dentin mineralization but not matrix formation; therefore, the architectural form of tubules remains unaffected. Peritubular dentin, however, is usually absent in these areas. Another area of dentin in root called Tome's granular layer (TGL) is also hypomineralized but usually less than IGD.

3.4.2 Key Identifying Features

IGD appears as irregular small cracks in the dentin. Their irregular borders indicate non-fusion of calcospherites. In ground sections, it usually appears dark and black due to the reflection of transmitted light from these uncalcified areas.

3.4.3 Clinical Significance

It is observed that IGD is more common in crowns than in the roots of teeth [8]. It appears as a consequence of irregularities in the globular pattern of mineralization leading to these hypomineralized areas of dentin [9]. The development of IGD has been noticed to increase during rickets and fluorosis [10, 11]. It has also been reported that retraction of the odontoblastic process from dentinal tubules could be involved in the development of IGD [8]. Considering its composition, it can be anticipated that dentin caries can spread through these areas at a much faster rate as compared to other parts due to the lack of mineralization.

3.5 Peritubular/Intratubular and Intertubular Dentin

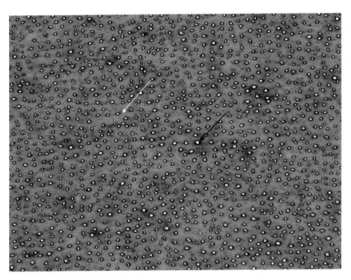

Figure 3.11 H and E stained section of dentin (black arrow, peritubular dentin; white arrow, intertubular dentin).

3.5.1 Description

Peritubular dentin or intratubular dentin is defined as the type of dentin that forms the covering of the dentinal tubules and also formulates the inner lining of tubules and thus surrounds the odontoblastic process. The dentin present between tubules is called intertubular dentin. The peritubular dentin is hypermineralized and contains fewer collagen fibers. It is estimated that peritubular dentin is 5–12% more mineralized than intertubular dentin, lacks a stabilizing collagen fiber network, and can easily be lost in routine demineralization cycles. Both these types are formed at almost the

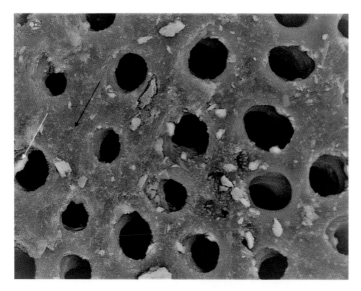

Figure 3.12 SEM image showing dentin (black arrow, intertubular dentin; white arrow, fractured peritubular dentin).

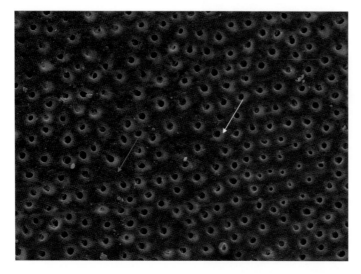

Figure 3.13 SEM image showing intertubular (blue arrow) and peritubular dentin (white arrow).

same time. The peritubular dentin covers more areas of outer dentin compared to tissue present near predentin and the microhardness and Young's modulus of the peritubular dentin is higher than intertubular dentin.

3.5.2 Key Identifying Features

The peritubular dentin forms a circular cuff or collar of dentin in a ring-like fashion around dentinal tubules on transverse sections. The intertubular dentin is present in the spaces between the adjacent tubules.

3.5.3 Clinical Significance

The peritubular dentin formation increases with age and thus the lumen size of dentinal tubule decreases [12]. This deposition of peritubular dentin is under the control of odontoblasts [7]. In addition, deposition of minerals inside the tubules in response to trauma or caries (called reactive dentin sclerosis) aids in the reduction of DH by decreasing the permeability of tubules [12]. It has also been proposed that the deposition of peritubular dentin leads to an increase in strength of outer dentin, especially in older patients [13]. The intertubular dentin is composed of mineralized collagen fibers (type I) and covers most of the area of dentin [14]. While performing composite restorations, monomer diffuses through the tubules (i.e. peritubular dentinal permeability) and through the intertubular dentin (intertubular dentinal permeability) [15]. Both of these are imperative in dentin bonding [15]. In fact, the area of intertubular dentin available for bonding is proportional to a resin restoration's surface adhesion [16].

3.6 Dead Tracts

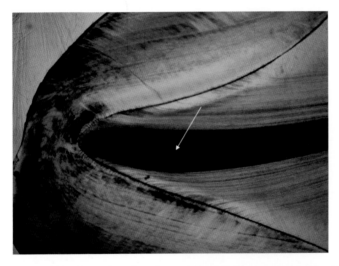

Figure 3.14 Ground section of enamel and dentin (arrow, dead tracts).

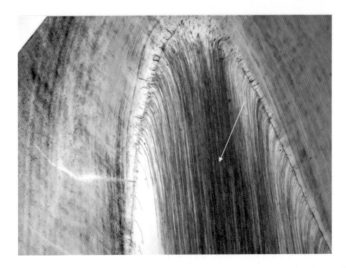

Figure 3.15 Ground section of enamel and dentin (arrow, dead tracts).

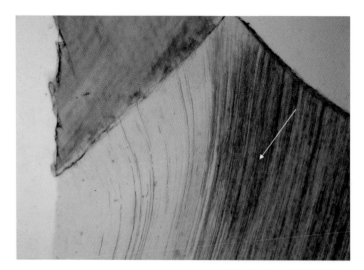

Figure 3.16 Ground section of enamel and dentin (arrow, dead tracts).

3.6.1 Description

Many tissues in the human body are reactive, which means that they respond to an external insult, and form a protective tissue. Dentin is an example of such a tissue and it forms dead tracts, tertiary dentin, and sclerotic dentin in response to external stimuli. Dentinal tubules usually contain dentinal fluid, odontoblastic process, and may contain sensory nerve terminals. Sometimes, these tubules are empty and get filled up by the air. These air-filled tubules when observed the under light microscope, appear darker in transmitted light than the regular tubules and are called dead tracts. The reason for these tubules to appear darker is the refraction of light from these air-confined tubules. The tubules can become empty because of the retraction of the odontoblastic process due to the carious process. In cases of trauma, if the primary odontoblasts are damaged, dead tracts are also formed.

3.6.2 Key Identifying Features

Dead tracts follow the same course of dentinal tubules but are darker in appearance than the regular dentinal tubules. A zone of tertiary dentin is usually seen beneath dead tracts which appears as a defensive mechanism. They appear black in transmitted while white in reflected light.

3.6.3 Clinical Significance

Fish gave the name dead tracts to air-filled tubules in the late 1920s [17]. Dead tracts could be defined as nonfunctional dentinal tubules [18]. It has been proposed that dead tracts appear because of an injury to terminal odontoblastic processes [19]. Trauma, erosion, attrition, and dental caries could all lead to the formation of dead tracts [20]. In normal teeth, dead tracts are also sometimes visible due to the degeneration of the odontoblastic processes during tooth development [21]. By definition, a true dead tract is the one which is surrounded by a cover of sclerotic (translucent) dentin [18].

3.7 Tertiary Dentin

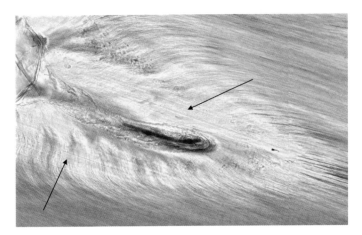

Figure 3.17 Ground section of enamel and dentin (arrows, tertiary dentin).

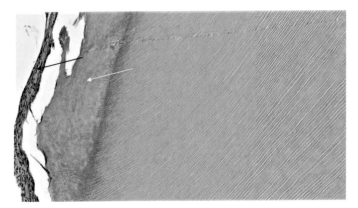

Figure 3.18 H and E stained decalcified section of regular and tertiary dentin (black arrow, pulp; white arrow, tertiary dentin).

3.7.1 Description

Tertiary dentin is formed in response to an external insult like trauma, attrition, abrasion, restorative procedure, or dental caries. Tertiary dentin has two types: reactionary and reparative. Reactionary tertiary dentin is formed in scenarios where odontoblasts become hyperplastic and deposit excess tissue in response to an external stimulus as a protective mechanism. This reactionary dentin has a tubular structure that is continuous with primary and secondary dentin. Reparative tertiary dentin is formed in cases where external trauma leads to death of odontoblasts. Undifferentiated cells from the pulp then change into new odontoblasts and secrete reparative tissue called reparative tertiary dentin. Dentinogenesis involving the formation of reactionary and reparative type is different as in the former, a simple upregulation in the activity of odontoblasts is required whereas the latter requires recruitment, differentiation, and enhancement of dentin development and deposition activity. If the odontoblast cells get trapped within the dentin, the tissue starts to resemble bone and is called osteodentin. This results from a quick rate of tertiary dentin formation. The quantity of tertiary dentin deposited is directly proportional to the intensity and duration of the stimulus. Dentinal tubules usually appear distorted and less organized in tertiary dentin, especially in the reparative type. Due to variation in its appearance, tertiary dentin is also sometimes called irregular secondary dentin.

3.7.2 Key Identifying Features

The dentin area with an irregular tubular pattern represents tertiary dentin and is usually seen toward the inside of the tooth in dentin adjacent to pulp. Cellular inclusions inside dentin can be seen in this type of dentin.

3.7.3 Clinical Significance

Formation of tertiary dentin is a protective mechanism of the pulp to protect itself from an insult such as trauma or caries [22]. This dentinal bridge over the pulp is more denser than regular dentin and protects it from the infecting bacteria and advancing carious lesion [23]. In clinical dentistry, the use of certain materials such as mineral trioxide aggregate (MTA) or calcium hydroxide for indirect or direct pulp capping procedures induces the formation of reactionary or reparative tertiary dentin [24]. In older individuals, secondary and tertiary dentin formation leads to a reduction in the size of the pulp chamber which can lead to a reduction in pulp vitality and sensitivity [25]. The evidence of occlusal attrition due to a long period of functioning is very common in older patients and can also lead to the formation of tertiary dentin [26].

3.8 Sclerotic Dentin

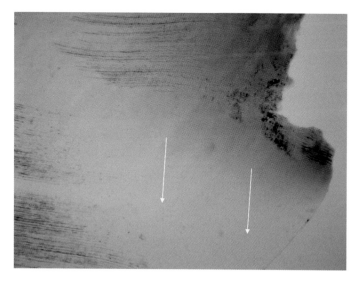

Figure 3.19 Ground section showing sclerotic dentin (arrows, translucent area in dentin representing sclerotic dentin).

3.8.1 Description

The word "sclerosis" means abnormal hardening of tissue. Sclerotic dentin is a type of dentin in which the tubules become occluded by minerals in response to stimuli such as a slowly progressing carious lesion or trauma like mild irritation. The tubules could be partially or sometimes completely occluded. The obliteration moves from the EDJ toward the pulp. It is a highly mineralized type of tissue in which the patency of the tubules is decreased as the mineral deposition increases. The tubules in sclerotic dentin become less permeable and transmit less stimuli. It appears as glassy or translucent in ground sections and is most commonly seen in the root areas. The deposition of sclerotic dentin increases with age (physiological dentin sclerosis) although it could occur in young age, as well as due to irritation (reactive dentin sclerosis). It is not clear whether this increased mineralization is due to a quantitative increase of mineral salts or hyper-mineralization of existing dentin.

3.8.2 Key Identifying Features

Sclerotic dentin appears bright, shiny, glassy, and translucent/transparent. Transverse sections of tubules could show decreased sized lumen of dentinal tubules due to mineral deposition. The reduction in size depends on the degree of mineralization.

3.8.3 Clinical Significance

The deposition of minerals and the resulting occlusion of dentinal tubules protect the pulp vitality and make it less sensitive [5]. This is supported by the fact that dental practitioners can usually proceed with dental procedures without local anesthesia administration in older patients [27]. It is believed that the hardness of sclerotic dentin is higher than normal dentin due to higher mineralization [28]. However, some studies have reported that its hardness under carious lesions is equal or sometimes less than intact dentin [29, 30]. Sclerotic dentin poses a challenge during placement of composite restorations especially when this hypermineralized layer is thick and a mild etchant is used [31].

3.9 Tome's Granular Layer (TGL)

3.9.1 Description

The TGL is also called the granular layer of Tomes, or granular dentin. It is visible microscopically on ground sections in the root area of teeth. On its outer side, cementum is visible. The TGL becomes more prominent with increased granules from the cervical region toward the apical area. TGL were initially thought to be hypomineralized areas, similar to IGD which appears due to non-fusion of calcospherites. However, the currently most accepted explanation defines TGL as area where dentinal tubules branch abundantly and loop back on themselves, creating air-filled spaces that appear granular when observed under transmitted light.

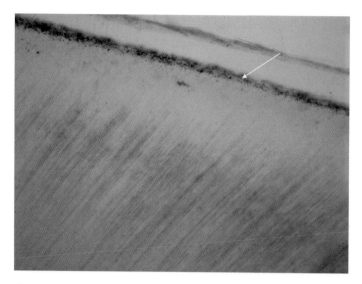

Figure 3.20 Ground section of root showing Tome's granular layer (arrow).

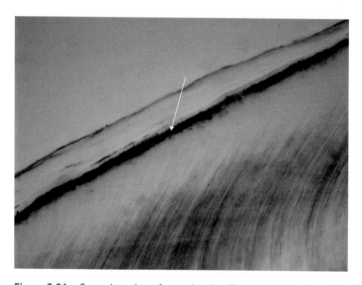

Figure 3.21 Ground section of root showing Tome's granular layer (arrow).

3.9.2 Key Identifying Features

This layer appears dark and black just adjacent to cementum under transmitted light toward the superficial surface of dentin. TGL is present in the root area, and only observed on ground sections, and cannot be seen on H and E stained sections of teeth. These granules are mostly parallel to each other and thus form the outer boundary of root dentin extending to the cementodentinal junction.

3.9.3 Clinical Significance

A previous study using Electron Probe Microanalysis has shown that the TGL is rich in calcium and phosphorus, more than IGD, and predentin (first formed dentin which is more organic and less mineralized) [32]. More calcium and phosphate implicates more resistance to carious attacks compared to IGD. The TGL can be variable in appearance in certain diseases, e.g. in cleidocranial dysostosis (CCD), it beceomes irregular [33], whereas its thickness increases in fluorosis-affected teeth [34]. The exact reason for these changes is still unclear.

3.10 Dentin Caries

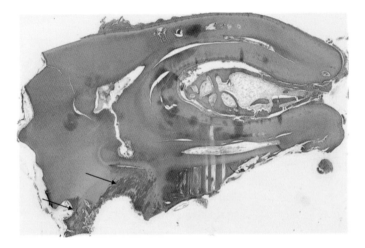

Figure 3.22 H and E stained section showing prominent dentin caries (arrows).

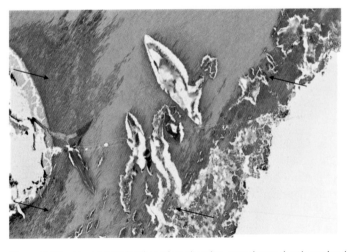

Figure 3.23 H and E stained section showing prominent dentin caries (arrows).

3.10.1 Description

Dental caries is a bacterial disease involving demineralization of the tooth structure by microorganism-derived organic acids resulting from fermentation of dietary carbohydrates. If the caries is not treated while it is restricted to the enamel, it can progress into dentin to cause dentinal caries. Caries in dentin can be "actively progressing" (soft and wet in clinical appearance) or "slowly progressing" (leathery or hard). These two types of dentin caries can interchange and actively progress. Dentinal caries traditionally is divided into five zones (from outside to inside) including zone of decomposed dentin, zone of bacterial invasion, zone of decalcification, zone of dentinal sclerosis, and zone of fatty degeneration. In the initial stages of dentin caries, minerals are dissolved without any effect on the collagen fibers which can colonize bacteria. However, at a more advanced progressive stage, even the collagen fibers are broken down by enzymes. It should be noted that the same level of acid exposure causes more significant caries in dentin compared to enamel due to its lower mineral content and smaller crystal size.

3.10.2 Key Identifying Features

On histological sections, disruption is seen in the tooth's outline due to dentinal caries in various focal areas. Numerous clefts which are usually perpendicular to the direction of dentinal tubules are also seen.

3.10.3 Clinical Considerations

Dental caries in dentin spreads faster than enamel as this tissue has lower mineral content [35]. Carious dentin has a low hardness and elastic modulus compared to the normal dentin [36]. The treatment of dentinal caries is the partial or complete excavation of the carious lesion, depending on its proximity with the pulp [37].

References

1 Ali, S. and Farooq, I. (2013). Dentine hypersensitivity: a review of its etiology, mechanism, prevention strategies and recent advancements in its management. *World J Dent* 4 (3): 188–192.

2 Lin, M., Luo, Z.Y., Bai, B.F. et al. (2011). Fluid mechanics in dentinal microtubules provides mechanistic insights into the difference between hot and cold dental pain. *PLoS One* 6 (3): e18068.

3 Farooq, I., Moheet, I.A., and AlShwaimi, E. (2015). In vitro dentine tubule occlusion and remineralization competence of various toothpastes. *Arch Oral Biol* 60 (9): 1246–1253.

4 Tomoaia, G. and Pasca, R.D. (2015). On the collagen mineralization. A review. *Clujul Med* 88 (1): 15–22.

5 Nanci, A. and Ten, C.A.R. (2003). *Ten Cate's Oral Histology: Development, Structure, and Function.* St. Louis: Mosby.

6 Mejàre, I. and Stenlund, H. (2000). Caries rates for the mesial surface of the first permanent molar and the distal surface of the second primary molar from 6 to 12 years of age in Sweden. *Caries Res* 34 (6): 454–461.

7 Mjör, I.A. (2009). Dentine permeability: the basis for understanding pulp reactions and adhesive technology. *Braz Dent J* 20 (1): 3–16.

8 Jayawardena, C., Nandasena, T., Abeywardena, A., and Nanayakkara, D. (2009). Regional distribution of interglobular dentinee in human teeth. *Arch Oral Biol* 54 (11): 1016–1021.

9 Avery, J.K. (2000). *Essentials of Oral Histology and Embryology*, 2e, 95–106. Missouri: Mosby.

10 Boukpessi, T., Septier, D., Bagga, S. et al. (2006). Dentine alteration of deciduous teeth in human hypophosphatemic rickets. *Calcif Tissue Int* 79 (5): 294–300.

11 Milan, A.M., Waddington, R.J., and Embery, G. (2001). Fluoride alters casein kinase II and alkaline phosphatase activity in vitro with potential implications for dentinee mineralization. *Arch Oral Biol* 46 (4): 343–351.

12 Tjäderhane, L. (2019). Dentine basic structure, composition, and function. In: *The Root Canal Anatomy in Permanent Dentition* (eds. M. Versiani, B. Basrani and M. Sousa-Neto). Cham: Springer.

13 Montoya, C., Arango-Santander, S., Peláez-Vargas, A. et al. (2015). Effect of aging on the microstructure, hardness and chemical composition of dentine. *Arch Oral Biol* 60 (12): 1811–1820.

14 Spencer, P., Ye, Q., Park, J. et al. (2010). Adhesive/Dentine interface: the weak link in the composite restoration. *Ann Biomed Eng* 38 (6): 1989–2003.

15 Kumar, J.S. and Jayalakshmi, S. (2016). Bond failure and its prevention in composite restoration: a review. *Pharm Sci Res* 8 (7): 627–631.

16 Pegado, R.E., do Amaral, F.L., Flório, F.M., and Basting, R.T. (2010). Effect of different bonding strategies on adhesion to deep and superficial permanent dentine. *Eur J Dent* 4 (2): 110–117.

17 Fish, E.W. (1928). Dead tracts in dentinee. *Proc R Soc Med* 22 (2): 227–236.

18 Chowdhary, N. and Subba Reddy, V.V. (2010). Dentine comparison in primary and permanent molars under transmitted and polarised light microscopy: an in vitro study. *J Indian Soc Pedod Prev Dent* 28: 167–172.

19 Fish, E.W. (1928). Physiology of dentine and its reaction to injury and disease. *Br Dent J* 49: 593.

20 Stanley, H.R., Pereica, J.C., Spiegel, E. et al. (1983). The detection and prevalence of reactive and physiologic, sclerotic dentine reparative and dead tracts beneath various types of dental lesions according to tooth surface and age. *J Oral Pathol* 12: 257–289.

21 Berkovitz (1995). *Dentine in Oral Anatomy and Embryology*, 130–143. Toronto, ON: Mosby.

22 Choung, H.W., Lee, D.S., Lee, J.H. et al. (2016). Tertiary dentine formation after indirect pulp capping using protein CPNE7. *J Dent Res* 95 (8): 906–912.

23 Smith, A.J., Cassidy, N., Perry, H. et al. (1995). Reactionary dentineogenesis. *Int J Dev Biol* 39 (1): 273–280.

24 Song, M., Yu, B., Kim, S. et al. (2017). Clinical and molecular perspectives of reparative dentine formation: lessons learned from pulp-capping materials and the emerging roles of calcium. *Dent Clin North Am* 61 (1): 93–110.

25 Johnstone, M. and Parashos, P. (2015). Endodontics and the ageing patient. *Aust Dent J* 60 (Suppl 1): 20–27.

26 Gustafson, G. (1950). Age determination on teeth. *J Am Dent Assoc* 41: 45–54.

27 Ghazali, F.B. (2003). Permeability of dentinee. *Malays J Med Sci* 10 (1): 27–36.

28 Martín, N., García, A., Vera, V. et al. (2010). Mechanical characterization of sclerotic occlusal dentine by nanoindentation and nanoscratch. *Am J Dent* 23 (2): 108–112.

29 Marshall, G.W., Habelitz, S., Gallagher, R. et al. (2001). Nanomechanical properties of hydrated carious human dentine. *J Dent Res* 80 (8): 1768–1771.

30 Ogawa, K., Yamashita, Y., Ichijo, T., and Fusayama, T. (1983). The ultrastructure and hardness of the transparent layer of human carious dentine. *J Dent Res* 62 (1): 7–10.

31 Tay, F.R. and Pashley, D.H. (2004). Resin bonding to cervical sclerotic dentine: a review. *J Dent* 32 (3): 173–196.

32 Tsuchiya, M., Sasano, Y., Kagayama, M., and Watanabe, M. (2001). Characterization of interglobular dentine and Tomes' granular layer in dog dentine using electron probe microanalysis in comparison with predentine. *Calcif Tissue Int* 68 (3): 172–178.

33 Fukuta, Y., Totsuka, M., Fukuta, Y. et al. (2001). Histological and analytical studies of a tooth in a patient with cleidocranial dysostosis. *J Oral Sci* 43 (2): 85–89.

34 Ramesh, M., Narasimhan, M., Krishnan, R. et al. (2017). The effect of fluorosis on human teeth under light microscopy: a cross-sectional study. *J Oral Maxillofac Pathol* 21 (3): 345–350.

35 Takahashi, N. and Nyvad, B. (2016). Ecological hypothesis of dentin and root caries. *Caries Res* 50 (4): 422–431.

36 Ito, S., Saito, T., Tay, F.R. et al. (2005). Water content and apparent stiffness of non-caries versus caries-affected human dentin. *J Biomed Mater Res B Appl Biomater* 72 (1): 109–116.

37 Thompson, V., Craig, R.G., Curro, F.A. et al. (2008). Treatment of deep carious lesions by complete excavation or partial removal: a critical review. *J Am Dent Assoc* 139 (6): 705–712.

4

Cementum

Saqib Ali¹, Imran Farooq¹, Amr Bugshan¹, Erum Khan²,³, and Syed Ali Khurram⁴

¹ Department of Biomedical Dental Sciences, College of Dentistry, Imam Abdulrahman Bin Faisal University, Dammam, Saudi Arabia
² CODE-M Center of Dental Education & Medicine, Karachi, Pakistan
³ Bhitai Dental and Medical College, Liaquat University of Medical and Health Sciences, Jamshoro, Pakistan
⁴ Unit of Oral and Maxillofacial Pathology, School of Clinical Dentistry, University of Sheffield, Sheffield, United Kingdom

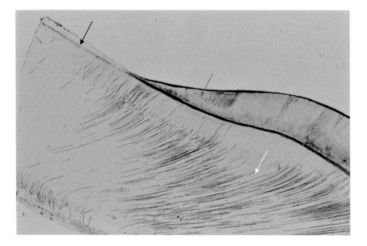

Figure 4.1 Ground section showing enamel (blue arrow), dentin (white arrow), and cementum (black arrow).

Cementum is mineralized tissue which covers the root of the teeth. It is secreted by cells called cementoblasts which are differentiated from the dental follicle. Anatomically, it is thinnest in the cervical region (20–50 μm) and its thickness increases toward the root apex (150–200 μm). It is a component of the periodontium, others being gingiva, periodontal ligament (PDL), and alveolar bone. The prime function of cementum is to provide an attachment to the PDL fibers. In addition, it also has a protective function for radicular dentin. Composition wise, it is less mineralized than enamel and dentin, and very similar in composition to the bone with approximately 65% inorganic material, 23% organic material, and 12% water. Inorganic component is composed of HAP crystals which are smaller than enamel and dentin but similar to those seen in bone. Organic material comprises mostly of type I collagen fibers with a few protein molecules. Because of its compositional resemblance to bone, cementum is sometimes also called as a modified bone but it should

An Illustrated Guide to Oral Histology, First Edition. Edited by Imran Farooq, Saqib Ali, and Paul Anderson.
© 2021 John Wiley & Sons Ltd. Published 2021 by John Wiley & Sons Ltd.
Companion website: www.wiley.com/go/farooq/oral_histology

be noted that cementum is avascular and aneural, unlike bone. Also, cementum has no lamellae (layers) like bone and is devoid of any marrow spaces. Cementum like other hard tissues is formed incrementally which leads to development of incremental lines (of Salter) evident in its structure. There are different types of cementum based on various classifications with the most popular classification dividing it into acellular (without cells) and cellular type. Incremental lines are closer in acellular type while they are wider apart in cellular cementum. Cementum is an important tooth component and its key features are discussed in the following sections.

4.1 Acellular Cementum

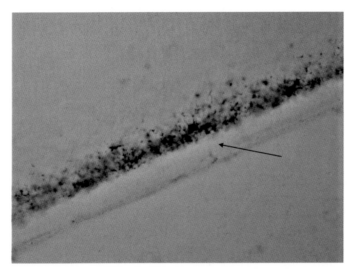

Figure 4.2   Ground section showing dentin and cementum (arrows, acellular cementum).

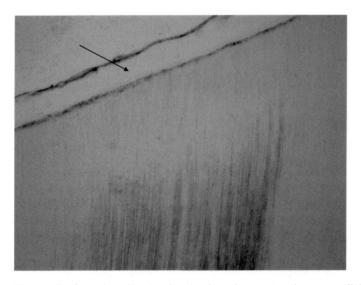

Figure 4.3   Ground section showing dentin and cementum (arrows, acellular cementum).

4.1.1   Description

Acellular cementum is the first formed cementum; this is why it is sometimes also called as primary cementum. It is formed more slowly than its counterpart, i.e. cellular cementum. As the name indicates, acellular contains no cells (cementocytes). Therefore, the incremental lines (of Salter) in this type of cementum are closer to each other. It is located at the cervical two-third of the root but is also present in apical one-third where cellular cementum overlaps it. It should be noted, however, that in certain individuals this arrangement is opposite, i.e. acellular overlaps cellular in apical one-third. Acellular cementum is present outside the Tome's granular layer (TGL) and it is difficult to differentiate it from the hyaline layer (which binds cementum with dentin). As this type of dentin is deficient in cells, it contains more minerals which make this structure highly mineralized compared to cellular cementum. Acellular cementum only contains extrinsic fibers which run perpendicular to the root surface.

4.1.2   Key Identifying Features

Acellular cementum appears structureless and lack cells, located toward the outer surface of tooth root. Its most common location is cervical two-third of the root and appears as clear tissue, just outside the TGL.

4.1.3   Clinical Significance

As acellular cementum is devoid of any cells, it does not have a reparative function [1]. The primary role of acellular cementum is to provide an attachment to PDL Sharpey fibers which help solidify the attachment apparatus as PDL fibers are inserted in cementum at one end and in alveolar bone at the other [2]. With regards to root restorations, numerous studies have been reported in the literature. Ferrari et al. reported that in resin restorations, the strength of the bond when applied to the cementum is unpredictable [3]. On the other hand, Van Dijken et al. reported admirable resin adaptation on cementum, especially below the cervical margins [4]. It is not clear whether this variation is due to variation in the structure of cementum or is due to different properties of bonding materials. Gingival recession causing exposure of cementum could result in its removal due to mechanical friction leading to DH [5].

4.2   Cellular Cementum

4.2.1   Description

Cellular cementum is formed after acellular cementum and is sometimes referred to as secondary cementum. It is formed quicker compared to acellular cementum. Cellular type contains cells called cementocytes which represent entrapped cementoblasts. The incremental lines in this type of cementum are farther apart from each other. It is predominantly seen in the apical one-third of the root where cellular cementum overlaps acellular cementum and is also common in inter-radicular/furcation areas. Due to the presence of cells, it contains less minerals making it less mineralized compared to acellular cementum. Cellular type could contain both extrinsic fibers (which run perpendicular to the root surface) and intrinsic fibers (which run parallel to the root surface).

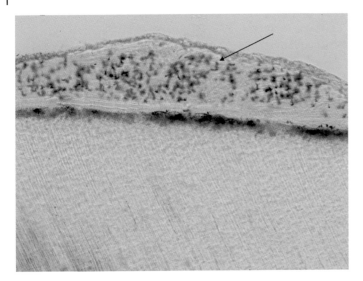

Figure 4.4 Ground section of cementum and dentin (arrow, cellular cementum).

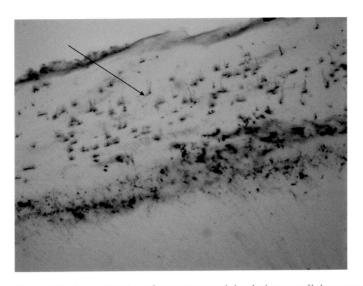

Figure 4.5 Ground section of cementum and dentin (arrow, cellular cementum).

As cementum is avascular, cementocytes are arranged randomly and dispersed throughout the tissue. This arrangement makes it different from osteocytes (bone cells) which are arranged circumferentially around blood vessels called haversian canals.

4.2.2 Key Identifying Features

Cellular cementum is found overlapping acellular cementum in the apical one-third of the tooth root. On ground sections, this tissue appears white with black dot-like areas indicating cementosteocytes.

4.2.3 Clinical Significance

As cellular cementum contains cells, it has a more reparative function [1]. Cellular cementum is able to repair itself to some extent but it cannot regenerate [6]. As with the normal aging process or due to orthodontic tooth movement, resorption can be seen in cellular cementum in the apical one-third of the tooth [7]. Cellular cementum tries to maintain continuous deposition in these cases to maintain integrity of the attachment apparatus [1].

4.3 Cementocytes and Lacunae

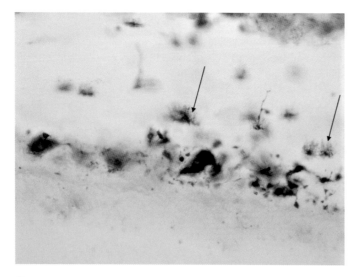

Figure 4.6 Ground section of cellular cementum (arrow, cementocytes lacunae with canaliculi).

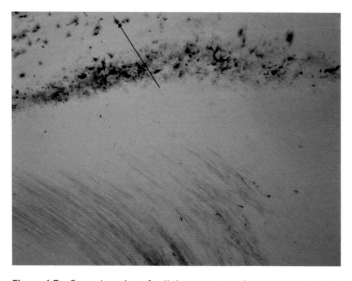

Figure 4.7 Ground section of cellular cementum (arrow, cementocyte lacunae with canaliculi).

4.3.1 Description

Cementocytes are cells present in cellular cementum and represent cementoblasts entrapped in their own matrix during mineralization losing the capability to secrete. The spaces occupied by cementocytes are called lacunae whereas their extensions are called canaliculi. Cementocyte lacunae are bigger in size compared to osteocyte lacunae and, therefore, can accommodate more than one cell. Unlike osteocytes whose life span is dependent on bony remodeling, the life span of a cementocyte is much longer as cementum is much less resorbable (especially in young age) and has less ability to repair itself.

4.3.2 Key Identifying Features

Cementocyte lacunae appear black in ground sections. These black areas appear during preparations of ground sections as cells are lost and their previously occupied spaces get filled up with air and debris which appear dark under microscope transmitted light.

4.3.3 Clinical Significance

The exact role of cementocytes is not established clearly in the literature. Osteocytes have been reported to be mechanosensor cells regulating bone homeostasis whereas the function of cementocytes is unclear [8]. It is speculated that these cells could have a role in cellular cementum formation but at present there is no evidence to support this hypothesis [9].

4.4 Cementoenamel Junction (CEJ)

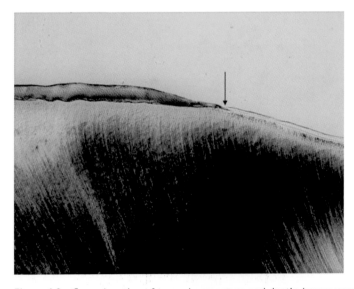

Figure 4.8 Ground section of enamel, cementum, and dentin (arrow, overlapping CEJ).

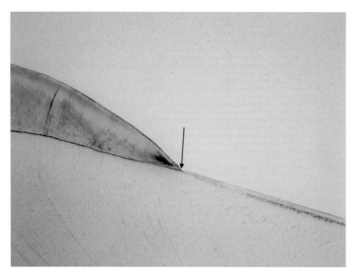

Figure 4.9 Ground section of enamel, cementum, and dentin (arrow, meeting CEJ).

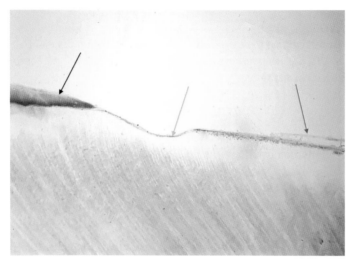

Figure 4.10 Ground section of enamel, cementum, and dentin (black arrow, enamel; blue arrow, cementum; orange arrow, gap between these two tissues).

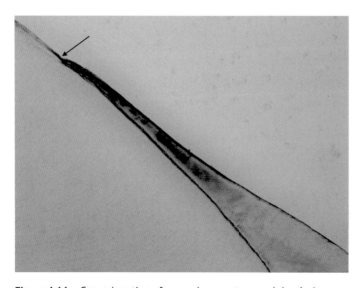

Figure 4.11 Ground section of enamel, cementum, and dentin (arrow, enamel overlapping cementum).

4.4.1 Description

The junction between cementum and enamel is called CEJ. This junction has three types which could be remembered as the OMG rule where: "O" indicates cementum *overlapping* enamel, "M" denotes cementum just *meeting* the enamel, and "G" indicates a small *gap* present between cementum and enamel. In the third type, the junction between cementum and enamel is actually absent due to the presence of the gap. Overlapping junction is most common and is present in 60–65% individuals followed by "meeting" junction which is present in approximately 30% individuals whereas gap junction is not very common and seen in only 10% of the cases. DH is very common in people with a gap junction. Another arrangement may also be present in few individuals where enamel is seen overlapping cementum. It should be noted however that all three types could be present in the same individual and even in the same tooth as CEJ is present on all sides of the tooth, i.e. buccal, mesial, palatal/lingual, and distal. This junction is not regular and usually has an irregular contour associated with it.

4.4.2 Key Identifying Features

The CEJ seen on ground sections shows enamel to be of brown color and cementum to be of pale or white color. Different patterns of CEJ are easily visible in the cervical margin area of the tooth, if cementum and enamel are identified correctly.

4.4.3 Clinical Significance

The CEJ is very important clinically as it demarcates where the crown ends and the anatomic root starts [10]. One example is periodontology where the extent of periodontal destruction is assessed by analyzing the loss of connective tissue attachment on tooth root, starting from CEJ [11]. The location of CEJ is considered a stationary landmark which can be used for clinical attachment loss (CAL) measurements and measurement of probing depths [12]. With increasing age, more of the CEJ could be exposed to the oral environment and thus could be subjected to a change because of the effect of various chemicals and oral hygiene products [12].

4.5 Hypercementosis

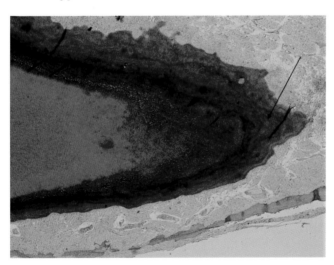

Figure 4.12 H and E stained decalcified section showing tooth apex (arrow, hypercementosis).

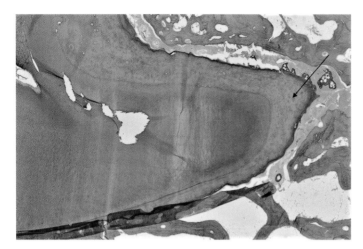

Figure 4.13 H and E stained decalcified section tooth apex (arrow, hypercementosis).

4.5.1 Description

The term hypercementosis indicates increased cementum formation and the presence of abnormally thickened cementum on the root surface. It can be caused by a number of factors including localized causes such as traumatic occlusion, dental trauma, and unopposed teeth as well as generalized causes including chronic periapical infections, Paget's disease (affecting all the teeth), acromegaly, and rheumatic fever.

4.5.2 Key Identifying Features

Increased thickness (more than usual) of cementum is seen around the tooth apex. It is an asymptomatic condition, mostly seen as an incidental finding on routine radiographs. Occasionally, in teeth with a previous history of trauma, there can be evidence of infraocclusion and hypercementosis.

4.5.3 Clinical Considerations

Hypercementosis can cause problems with tooth extraction particularly where ankylosis or concrescence (fusion of the roots) has taken place [13]. The differential diagnosis of hypercementosis includes condensing osteitis and cementoblastoma [14]. This increased cementum formation is a challenge for endodontic therapy as the canals could actually be located above the radiographic apex [15]. It has also been reported that hypercementosis can cause modification of the original path of the root canals, making endodontic treatment difficult [16]. Furthermore, hypercementosis could provide supplementary sites for the bacterial colonization, ultimately resulting in periapical periodontitis [17].

4.6 Cementoblastoma

4.6.1 Description

Cementoblastoma is a benign tumor derived from cementum. It is of odontogenic origin and usually there is no paresthesia of the associated teeth. It is considered as a true cemental neoplasm. Cementoblastoma has a predilection for males and is seen more commonly in mandibular

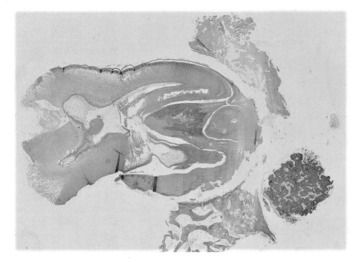

Figure 4.14 H and E stained decalcified section showing cementoblastoma associated with tooth root.

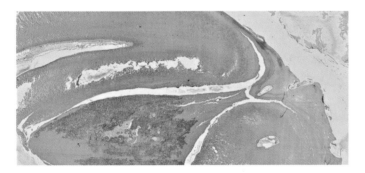

Figure 4.15 H and E stained decalcified section showing cementoblastoma associated with tooth root.

posterior teeth (premolars and molars). This tumor is usually asymptomatic and the pulp of the involved tooth is vital. Cementoblastoma mostly involves permanent teeth although it can rarely be seen in association with deciduous teeth.

4.6.2 Key Identifying Features

It appears as a calcified mass on histological sections and radiographs which is attached to the affected tooth roots. This mass appears to be fused with the tooth root and there is characteristically noticeable cementoblastic rimming.

4.6.3 Clinical Considerations

Cementoblastoma is an odontogenic tumor which has an incidence rate of less than 1% [18]. It is connected to the root of the affected tooth [19] and the patient typically presents with a swelling [20]. The differential diagnosis includes osteoblastoma which lacks attachment to the tooth root [21]. The treatment of choice is conservative removal of the tumor along with the tooth [22].

Recurrence is common and a recurrence rate as high as 37.1% has been reported in the literature [23]. The most common reason for the recurrence is incomplete surgical excision, leaving behind part of lesional tissue [24].

4.7 Root Resorption

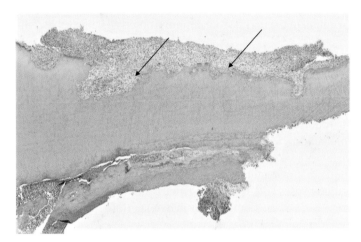

Figure 4.16 H and E stained decalcified section showing tooth root with prominent external resorption (arrows).

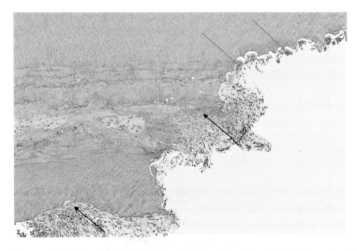

Figure 4.17 H and E stained decalcified section showing tooth root with prominent external resorption (black arrows) and multinucleated odontoclasts (blue arrows).

4.7.1 Description

Tooth root resorption involves resorption of cementum followed by dentin. It is carried out by a variant of osteoclasts called odontoclasts. It is a normal physiological process that occurs in the roots of primary teeth due to the pressure exerted by the permanent tooth as part of eruption and shedding. In permanent teeth, however, root resorption is usually caused by a pathological condition. Root resorption is mainly divided into two types: external and internal. The main causes of external root resorption in permanent teeth include excessive orthodontic forces, pulpal necrosis, trauma, cysts, tumors, and intra-coronal bleaching. Internal root resorption has an unknown etiology.

4.7.2   Key Identifying Features

On histological sections, a clear disruption of the normal root outline is observed with visible clefts toward the external surface.

4.7.3   Clinical Considerations

Root resorption does not occur during every orthodontic treatment. It is proposed that heavy orthodontic forces cause more resorption than light forces [25, 26] and compressive forces are more likely to cause root resorption compared to tensile forces [27]. Another important factor is the time period for which the active forces are applied, i.e. longer time leads to more resorption and vice versa [28]. To prevent orthodontic root resorption, light intermittent forces should be applied for longer durations between activation phases [29]. Certain systemic conditions such as hypoparathyroidism, hyperparathyroidism, Paget's disease, hypophosphatemia, Goltz syndrome, and Turner syndrome have also been reported to cause root resorption [30].

References

1 Yamamoto, T., Hasegawa, T., Yamamoto, T. et al. (2016). Histology of human cementum: its structure, function, and development. *Jpn Dent Sci Rev* 52 (3): 63–74.
2 LeBlanc, A.R. and Reisz, R.R. (2013). Periodontal ligament, cementum, and alveolar bone in the oldest herbivorous tetrapods, and their evolutionary significance. *PLoS One* 8 (9): e74697.
3 Ferrari, M., Cagidiago, M.C., and Davidson, C. (1997). Resistance of cementum in class II and V cavities to penetration by an adhesive system. *Dent Mater* 13: 157–162.
4 Van Dijken, J.W.V., Horsted, T.P., and Waern, R. (1998). Directed polymerization shrinkage versus a horizontal incremental technique: interfacial adaptation in vivo in class II cavities. *Am J Dent* 11: 165–172.
5 Davari, A., Ataei, E., and Assarzadeh, H. (2013). Dentine hypersensitivity: etiology, diagnosis and treatment; a literature review. *J Dent (Shiraz)* 14 (3): 136–145.
6 Bosshardt, D.D. and Schroeder, H.E. (1996). Cementogenesis reviewed: a comparison between human premolars and rodent molars. *Anat Rec* 245 (2): 267–292.
7 Feller, L., Khammissa, R.A., Thomadakis, G. et al. (2016). Apical external root resorption and repair in orthodontic tooth movement: biological events. *Biomed Res Int* 2016: 4864195.
8 Zhao, N., Foster, B.L., and Bonewald, L.F. (2016). The cementocyte-an osteocyte relative? *J Dent Res* 95 (7): 734–741.
9 Berkovitz, B.K.B., Holland, G.R., and Moxham, B.J. (2009). *Oral Anatomy, Histology and Embryology*. Edinburgh: Mosby/Elsevier.
10 Ceppi, E., Dall'Oca, S., Rimondini, L. et al. (2006). Cementoenamel junction of deciduous teeth: SEM-morphology. *Eur J Paediatr Dent* 7 (3): 131–134.

11 Preshaw, P.M., Kupp, L., Hefti, A.F., and Mariotti, A. (1999). Measurement of clinical attachment levels using a constant-force periodontal probe modified to detect the cemento-enamel junction. *J Clin Periodontol* 26 (7): 434–440.

12 Vandana, K.L. and Haneet, R.K. (2014). Cementoenamel junction: an insight. *J Indian Soc Periodontol* 18 (5): 549–554.

13 Palermo, D. and Davies-House, A. (2016). Unusual finding of concrescence. *BMJ Case Rep* 2016: bcr2016214597.

14 Weinberger, A. (1954). The clinical significance of hypercementosis. *Oral Surg Oral Med Oral Pathol* 7 (1): 79–87.

15 Pinheiro, B.C., Novaes, T., Capelozza, A.L.A., and Consolaro, A. (2008). A scanning electron microscopic study of hypercementosis. *J Appl Oral Sci* 16 (6): 380–384.

16 Fernanda, G.P., Cecilia, D.F., Jceue, M., and Luiz, F.M.S. (2011). Hypercementosis: a challenge for endodontic therapy. *RSBO* 8 (3): 321–328.

17 Zehnder, M., Gold, S.I., and Hasselgren, G. (2002). Pathologic interactions in pulpal and periodontal tissues. *J Clin Periodontol* 29 (8): 663–671.

18 Ulmansky, M., Hjørting-Hansen, E., Praetorius, F., and Haque, M.F. (1994). Benign cementoblastoma. A review and five new cases. *Oral Surg Oral Med Oral Pathol* 77 (1): 48–55.

19 Vieira, A.P., Meneses, J.M. Jr., and Maia, R.L. (2007). Cementoblastoma related to a primary tooth: a case report. *J Oral Pathol Med* 36: 117–119.

20 Slootweg, P.J. (1992). Cementoblastoma and osteoblastoma: a comparison of histological features. *J Oral Pathol Med* 21: 385–389.

21 Huber, A.R. and Folk, G.S. (2009). Cementoblastoma. *Head Neck Pathol* 3 (2): 133–135.

22 Sharma, N. (2014). Benign cementoblastoma: a rare case report with review of literature. *Contemp Clin Dent* 5 (1): 92–94.

23 Brannon, R.B., Fowler, C.B., Carpenter, W.M., and Corio, R.L. (2002). Cementoblastoma: an innocuous neoplasm? A clinicopathologic study of 44 cases and review of the literature with special emphasis on recurrence. *Oral Surg Oral Med Oral Pathol Oral Radiol Endod* 93: 311–320.

24 Sankari, L.S. and Ramakrishnan, K. (2011). Benign cementoblastoma. *J Oral Maxillofac Pathol* 15 (3): 358–360.

25 Harris, D.A., Jones, A.S., and Darendeliler, M.A. (2006). Physical properties of root cementum: part 8. Volumetric analysis of root resorption craters after application of controlled intrusive light and heavy orthodontic forces: a microcomputed tomography scan study. *Am J Orthod Dentofacial Orthop* 130: 639–647.

26 Barbagallo, L.J., Jones, A.S., Petocz, P., and Darendeliler, M.A. (2008). Physical properties of root cementum: part 10. Comparison of the effects of invisible removable thermoplastic appliances with light and heavy orthodontic forces on premolar cementum. Amicrocomputed-tomography study. *Am J Orthod Dentofacial Orthop* 133: 218–227.

27 Chan, E. and Darendeliler, M.A. (2006). Physical properties of root cementum: part 7. Extent of root resorption under areas of compression and tension. *Am J Orthod Dentofacial Orthop* 129: 504–510.

28 Segal, G., Shiffman, P., and Tuncay, O. (2004). Meta analysis of the treatment related factors of external apical root resorption. *Orthod Craniofacial Res* 7: 71–78.

29 Weltman, B., Vig, K.W.L., Fields, H.W. et al. (2010). Root resorption associated with orthodontic tooth movement: a systematic review. *Am J Orthod Dentofacial Orthop* 137: 462–476.

30 Khojastepour, L., Bronoosh, P., and Azar, M. (2010). Multiple idiopathic apical root resorption: a case report. *J Dent (Tehran)* 7 (3): 165–169.

5

Dental Pulp

Juzer Shabbir[1], Imran Farooq[2], Saqib Ali[2], Faraz Mohammed[2], Amr Bugshan[2], Syed Ali Khurram[3], and Erum Khan[4,5]

[1] Department of Operative Dentistry and Endodontics, Liaquat College of Medicine and Dentistry, Karachi, Pakistan
[2] Department of Biomedical Dental Sciences, College of Dentistry, Imam Abdulrahman Bin Faisal University, Dammam, Saudi Arabia
[3] Unit of Oral and Maxillofacial Pathology, School of Clinical Dentistry, University of Sheffield, Sheffield, United Kingdom
[4] CODE-M Center of Dental Education & Medicine, Karachi, Pakistan
[5] Bhitai Dental and Medical College, Liaquat University of Medical and Health Sciences, Jamshoro, Pakistan

Dental pulp is a soft tissue which is present inside the tooth and contains blood vessels, nerves, and lymphatics. It is present in both coronal and radicular portion of the tooth as shown in Figure 5.1.

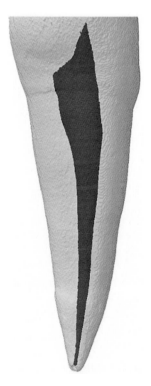

Figure 5.1 Micro-CT image showing dental pulp.

An Illustrated Guide to Oral Histology, First Edition. Edited by Imran Farooq, Saqib Ali, and Paul Anderson.
© 2021 John Wiley & Sons Ltd. Published 2021 by John Wiley & Sons Ltd.
Companion website: www.wiley.com/go/farooq/oral_histology

In terms of composition, it is 75% water and 25% of it is composed of organic material. The organic component of dental pulp is composed of collagen type I (60%) and type III (40%). In the organic composition, it is composed of protein molecules like versican, syndecan, decorin, and glycoproteins. The dental pulp is composed of cells which fall into four major categories, i.e. synthetic cells (odontoblasts and fibroblasts), progenitor cells (undifferentiated mesenchymal cells), defense cells (macrophages, lymphocytes, mast cells, etc.), and other cells (stem cells). The pulp forms an intimate bond with the dentin as odontoblast cell bodies are positioned in the pulp and their processes are present within the dentinal tubules. This relationship is sometimes referred to as pulpo-dentin complex. With increasing age, the size, number of cells, and vitality of the pulp decreases. Secondary dentin formation can take place on any surface of the pulp which leads to decreased pulp size. Hence in older patients, the pulp can appear narrow or obliterated on radiographs. The nerve fibers of pulp are responsible for transmitting dental pain, where alpha beta (a-β) and alpha delta (a-δ) fibers are responsible for sharp pain of short duration and C-fibers are accountable for transmitting dull throbbing pain of longer duration. The pulp has four histological zones, i.e. odontoblastic zone, cell-free zone of Weil, cell-rich zone, and pulp core (moving from outside to inside). These zones along with their contents and few pulpal pathologies are discussed in detail in the following sections.

5.1 Odontogenic Zone

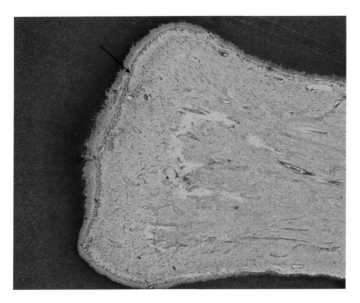

Figure 5.2 H and E stained decalcified section showing dentin and dental pulp (arrow, odontogenic zone).

5.1.1 Description

The odontogenic zone consists of cell bodies of columnar odontoblastic cells and their cytoplasmic processes. The characteristics of these cells may vary according to location. They have been found to vary from tall, pseudostratified columnar cells in the coronal area to a more cuboidal morphology in the radicular pulp. The cell bodies containing a large nucleus adjacent to the basement membrane make up the odontogenic zone, whereas its processes are positioned in the predentin matrix. The unmyelinated nerve fibers, capillaries, and dendritic cells can be found accompanying the odontoblast cells. These cells originate from peripheral mesenchymal cells of dental papilla during tooth development and differentiate by acquisition of distinctive morphology of glycoprotein synthesis and secretion. The collagen fibers have been shown to possess arrangement in a corkscrew-like fashion and are called "Von Korff's fibers." These fibers originate between odontoblasts and project into the dentin matrix. The odontoblastic processes are present in canaliculi which extend into the dentin layer and these canaliculi are called "dentinal tubules." In predentin, the odontoblastic processes run in compartments delimited by non-mineralized collagen fibers. There are approximately 59 000–76 000 dentinal tubules/mm^2 at the pulpal surface of the young premolar and molar crowns, whereas roughly half of this number is present near the enamel surface.

5.1.2 Key Identifying Features

The odontoblastic layer can be identified on histological sections as cellular (columnar) layer immediately below predentin and above the cell-free zone.

5.1.3 Clinical Significance

In a normal tooth, the first type of cells encountered when the pulp is approached are the odonto-blastic cells in the odontogenic zone [1]. Ultrastructural studies show that there are cytoplasmic networks between the odontoblasts and the subjacent mesenchymal cells and these connections serve to send signals to these undifferentiated mesenchymal cells upon injury [2]. The mesenchy-mal cells then proliferate and differentiate to become odontoblasts [2]. The odontoblasts lay down primary dentin till root formation is completed, whereas the secondary dentin is deposited post-root formation, in a similar manner to primary dentin [3]. Secondary dentin can be differentiated histologically from primary dentin by a subtle demarcation line, slight difference in staining, and less organized dental tubules [4].

5.2 Cell-Free Zone of Weil

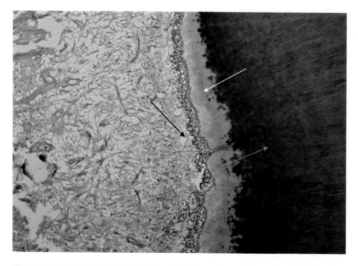

Figure 5.3 H and E stained decalcified section of dental pulp (black arrow, cell-free zone; white arrow, predentin; blue arrow, dentin).

5.2.1 Description

The cell-free zone of Weil is also called "sub-odontoblastic layer" or "Hoehl's layer." It is located below the odontoblastic layer and contains ramification of small nerve fibers (axons) and plexus' of capillaries. The cell-free and cell-rich zones can only be found in specific areas of the tooth and as the name indicated, the former contains a minimal number of cells.

5.2.2 Key Identifying Features

The cell-free zone of Weil can be identified on histological section as somewhat clear and sparsely cellular layer immediately below the odontogenic zone and above the cell-rich zone.

5.2.3 Clinical Significance

The cell-free zone layer serves to support both the cell-rich zone and the stratified odontoblastic layer [1]. The cell-free and cell-rich zones are typically indiscernible or missing in the embryonic pulp and they appear when dentin formation becomes active [4]. These zones become progressively more noticeable with the advancement of age and are less continuous and less protuberant at the apical area [1].

5.3 Cell-Rich Zone

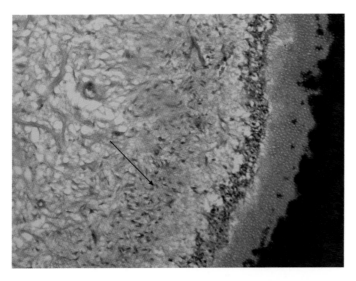

Figure 5.4 H and E stained section of dental pulp (arrow, cell-rich zone).

5.3.1 Description

This zone has a high cell density and can be easily seen in the coronal pulp. The cell-rich zone lies next to pulpal core and blends with it. Numerous fibroblast cells along with undifferentiated cells are seen in this zone. The number and shape of these fibroblasts depend on the age of the pulp. The pulpal fibroblast cells are spindle shaped, with ovoid nuclei and are responsible for synthesis and secretion of the bulk of extracellular components, i.e. collagen and ground substance.

5.3.2 Key Identifying Features

The cell-rich zone can be identified on histological section as a densely packed cellular layer above the pulpal core and below the cell-free zone.

5.3.3 Clinical Significance

The function of fibroblasts is to form and maintain pulp matrix [4]. In the cell-rich zone, the undifferentiated cells help in maintaining the quantity of odontoblasts by proliferation and differentiation [5]. Under appropriate stimulation, the undifferentiated mesenchymal cells (which are present adjacent to blood vessels) can distinguish into fixed or wandering histiocytes as well [6].

5.4 Pulp Core

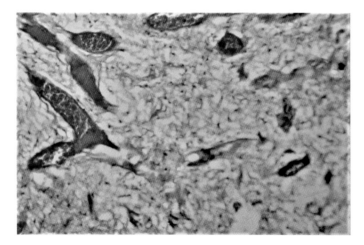

Figure 5.5 H and E stained section of dental pulp showing blood vessels in pulp core.

5.4.1 Description

The pulp core zone comprises prominent blood vessels and nerves and is present below the cell-rich zone. It consists mainly of ground substance which is an amorphous hydrated matrix gel and collagen fibrils. The ground substance is similar to other areolar, fibrous connective tissues primarily comprising protein complexes with a combination of glycosaminoglycans such as hyaluronic acid, chondroitin sulfate, as well as other glycoproteins, carbohydrates, and water. Collagen fibers in the pulp are unorganized and dispersed. Fibroblasts, undifferentiated mesenchymal cells (reserve cells), histiocytes, macrophages, polymorphonuclear leukocytes, lymphocytes, and mast cells are also present in this zone.

5.4.2 Key Identifying Features

Pulpal core can be identified on the histological section as loosely bound tissue in the center of the pulp below the cell-rich zone and shows a complex of blood vessels and nerves.

5.4.3 Clinical Significance

The combination of amorphous hydrated matrix gel and collagen fibrils in the pulpal core surrounds and supports pulpal cells and their sensory and vascular components [4]. The branches of the blood vessels and nerves in the pulpal core communicate with the critical outer layers of the pulp [4]. The matrix gel is similar to interstitial fluid, which acts like a transfer medium for nutrients and by-products between distantly separated cells of pulpal core and vasculature [1].

5.5 Pulpal Fibrosis

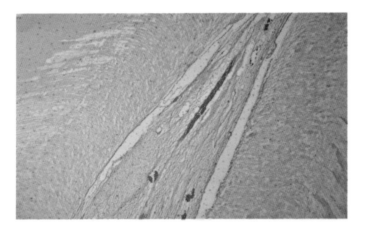

Figure 5.6   H and E stained section showing pulpal fibrosis.

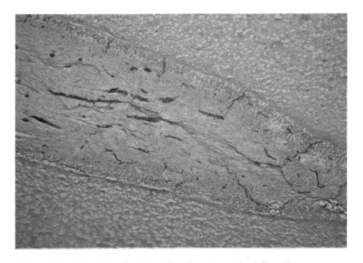

Figure 5.7   H and E stained section showing pulpal fibrosis.

5.5.1 Description

Pulp fibrosis is an age-related condition in which the pulp gets gradually replaced by fibrous bundles of collagen with aging. The pulp changes from loose to dense fibrous tissue and reduction of pulp volume with age favors this change. In some cases, the pulp may respond to irritating stimuli through accumulation of large collagenous fiber bundles. The dental pulp undergoes continual and slow compression due to continuous formation of secondary dentin. Radicular pulp has a smaller volume compared to coronal pulp; therefore, the physiologic compression is greater in the coronal pulp. This results in enhanced macromolecular crowding and excluded volume effect. This explains the increased fibrosis and arrangement of collagen fibers in bundles in radicular pulp compared to more diffuse deposition in the coronal pulp.

5.5.2 Key Identifying Features

It is represented by an increased number of collagen fibers (mostly in radicular pulp) and fewer number of cells.

5.5.3 Clinical Considerations

With increasing age, the pulp response time increases and pain intensity decreases due to physiological fibrosis [7]. Observing a degree of fibrosis (scarring) due to the conversion of loose connective tissue into a dense fibrous tissue is not uncommon [8].

5.6 Pulp Stones

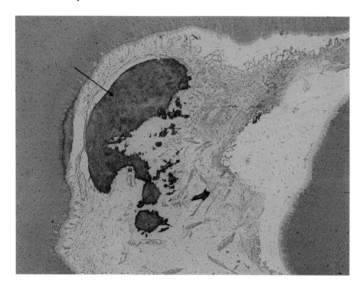

Figure 5.8 Decalcified H and E stained section of pulp (arrow, pulp stone).

5.6.1 Description

Pulp stones are discrete calcific masses having calcium–phosphorus ratios similar to that of dentin and are also called denticles. They may exist in isolation or in multiple numbers in any tooth. They

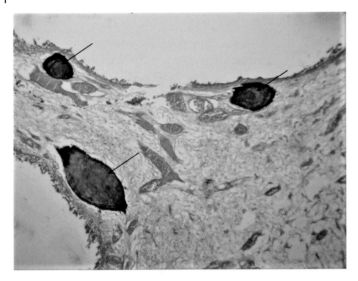

Figure 5.9 H and E stained section of pulp (arrows, pulp stones).

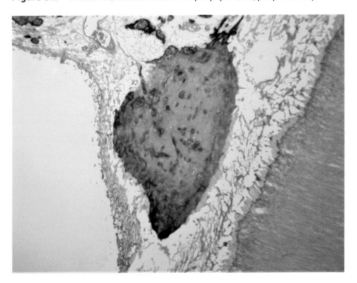

Figure 5.10 H and E stained section showing a pulp stone.

are most commonly located at the orifice of the pulp chamber or within the root canal. Pulp stones can be classified on the basis of their structure and location. On structural basis, they could be true or false pulp stones. True pulp stones are rare and comprise a central cavity with remnants of epithelial cells, may contain tubules, and could be surrounded by odontoblasts-like cells. Such stones have been reported to be present near the apex of the tooth. False pulp stones on the other hand do not have any particular associated cells. These are formed because of mineralization of degenerating pulpal cells. On the basis of location, denticles could be divided into (i) Free denticles, which are surrounded entirely by pulp and are not associated with dentin; (ii) Adherent, which are partly attached to the dentin; and (iii) Embedded, which are entirely surround by the dentin. True and free pulpal stones are commonly found in teeth with incomplete root formation. In teeth with fully developed roots, the stones are attached or embedded entirely in the dentinal wall.

5.6.2 Key Identifying Features

Pulp stones are seen in histological sections as darkly stained discrete masses within the core of the pulp. In histologic section, they usually possess characteristic concentric layer of mineralized tissue. In older teeth, pulp stones may contain atubular or tubular dentin surrounded by fibrodentin.

5.6.3 Clinical Considerations

Pulp stones usually grow as layers of mineralized tissue, formed by accumulation around dead or degenerating cells, collagen fibers, or blood thrombi [9]. A tooth may have single or multiple stones of fluctuating sizes (from minute to large), which can result in occlusion of pulpal space [9]. Pulp stones have been observed in patients with systemic or genetic diseases like dentin dysplasia, dentinogenesis imperfecta, and Van der Woude syndrome [10]. However, the exact cause of the presence of these stones is not completely known. Mandibular teeth have a higher incidence of pulp stones with first molars being most commonly affected [11]. These stones are known to offer difficulty in endodontic access to root canals and their shaping while root canal treatment [1, 12]. If required, pulp stones can be sectioned out of the access cavity by burs or by ultrasonic tips [13]. The usage of ultrasonic tips and sodium hypochlorite has synergistic effect on removal of these stones [14].

5.7 Periapical Granuloma

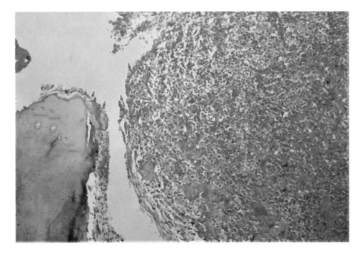

Figure 5.11 H and E stained section of tooth showing granulation tissue attached to the root apex with the features of mixed inflammatory cell infiltrates.

5.7.1 Description

Periapical granuloma is a consequence of pulpitis leading to the formation of granulation tissue at the root apex (periapical – around the apex). The affected tooth is non-vital but relatively asymptomatic. However, in the event of inflammation and as a result of swelling, the tooth becomes percussion-sensitive and when solid food is chewed, severe pain can be experienced. It is frequently identified in radiographs as a well-defined radiolucency, often less than 2 cm in size.

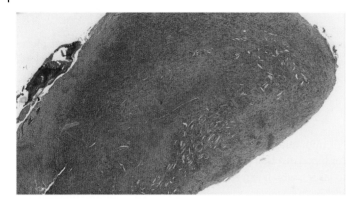

Figure 5.12 Low-power view of inflamed and vascular granulation tissue with denser fibrous tissue toward the periphery.

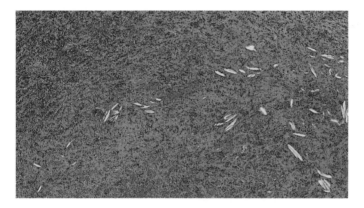

Figure 5.13 High-power view of granulation tissue containing chronic inflammatory cells and cholesterol clefts.

5.7.2 Key Identifying Features

Histopathologically, periapical granuloma comprises granulation tissue attached to the root apex containing a mixed inflammatory cell infiltrate comprising a few polymorphonuclear leukocytes with abundant lymphocytes, plasma cells, and histiocytes. Occasional giant cells, cholesterol clefts, Russel bodies (collection of gamma globulins produced by plasma cells) and scattered epithelial rests of Malassez can also be seen in granulation tissue.

5.7.3 Clinical Considerations

Histologically, a clinically diagnosed acute apical periodontitis may be classified as an acutely aggravated periapical granuloma, whereas a periapical abscess can progress to a periapical granuloma [15]. If left untreated, they can grow large, progress into a periapical/radicular cyst, or become acutely infected [16].

References

1 Pashley, D.H., Walton, R.E., and Slavkin, H.C. (2002). Histology and physiology of the dental pulp. In: *Endodontics*, 5e (eds. J.I. Ingle and L.K. Bakl), 25–60. Hamilton: BC Decker Inc.

2 Baume, L.J. (1980). *The Biology of Pulp and Dentine: A Historic, Terminologic-Taxonomic, Histologic-Biochemical, Embryonic and Clinical Survey*, Monographs in Oral Science, vol. 8, 123–141. New York: Karger.

3 Goldberg, M., Kulkarni, A.B., Young, M., and Boskey, A. (2011). Dentin: structure, composition and mineralization. *Front Biosci (Elite Ed)* 3: 711–735.

4 Nanci, A. (ed.) (2018). Dentin-pulp complex. In: *Ten Cate's Oral Histology: Development, Structure, and Function*, 9e. Missouri: Elsevier.

5 Bansal, R. and Jain, A. (2015). Current overview on dental stem cells applications in regenerative dentistry. *J Nat Sci Biol Med* 6 (1): 29–34.

6 Jean, A., Kerebel, B., and Kerebel, L.M. (1986). Scanning electron microscope study of the predentin-pulpal border zone in human dentin. *Oral Surg Oral Med Oral Pathol* 61 (4): 392–398.

7 Farac, R.V., Morgental, R.D., Lima, R.K. et al. (2012). Pulp sensibility test in elderly patients. *Gerodontology* 29 (2): 135–139.

8 Abbott, P.V. and Yu, C. (2007). A clinical classification of the status of the pulp and the root canal system. *Aust Dent J* 52 (1 Suppl): S17–S31.

9 Johnson, P.L. and Bevelander, G. (1956). Histogenesis and histochemistry of pulpal calcification. *J Dent Res* 35 (5): 714–722.

10 Kantaputra, P.N., Sumitsawan, Y., Schutte, B.C., and Tochareontanaphol, C. (2002). Van der Woude syndrome with sensorineural hearing loss, large craniofacial sinuses, dental pulp stones, and minor limb anomalies: report of a four-generation Thai family. *Am J Med Genet* 108 (4): 275–280.

11 Baghdady, V.S., Ghose, L.J., and Nahoom, H.Y. (1988). Prevalence of pulp stones in a teenage Iraqi group. *J Endod* 14 (6): 309–311.

12 Ibarrola, J.L., Knowles, K.I., Ludlow, M.O., and McKinley, I.B. Jr. (1997). Factors affecting the negotiability of second mesiobuccal canals in maxillary molars. *J Endod* 23 (4): 236–238.

13 Stamos, D.G., Haasch, G.C., Chenail, B., and Gerstein, H. (1985). Endosonics: clinical impressions. *J Endod* 11 (4): 181–187.

14 Cunningham, W.T. and Balekjian, A.Y. (1980). Effect of temperature on collagen-dissolving ability of sodium hypochlorite endodontic irrigant. *Oral Surg Oral Med Oral Pathol* 49 (2): 175–177.

15 Regezi, J.A. and Sciubba, J.J. (2008). *Oral Pathology: Clinical Pathologic Correlations*, 3e, 452–453. Philadelphia, New York: W. B. Saunders Company.

16 Krithika, C., Kota, S., Gopal, K.S., and Koteeswaran, D. (2011). Mixed periapical lesion: differential diagnosis of a case. *Dentomaxillofac Radiol* 40 (3): 191–194.

6

Periodontal Ligament

Saqlain Gilani[1], Imran Farooq[2], Saqib Ali[2], and Syed Ali Khurram[3]

[1] Department of Oral Biology, Islamic International Dental College, Riphah International University, Islamabad, Pakistan
[2] Department of Biomedical Dental Sciences, College of Dentistry, Imam Abdulrahman Bin Faisal University, Dammam, Saudi Arabia
[3] Unit of Oral and Maxillofacial Pathology, School of Clinical Dentistry, University of Sheffield, Sheffield, United Kingdom

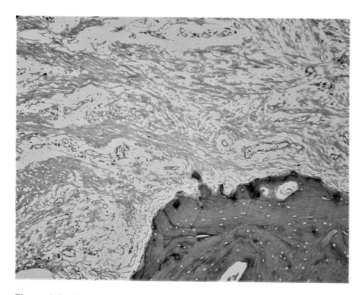

Figure 6.1 H and E stained section showing periodontal ligament (PDL) fibers radiating from bone.

The periodontium is comprised of two hard tissues (cementum and alveolar bone) and two soft tissues (gingiva and PDL). The PDL is a fibrous connective tissue which is present in all teeth. It fills up the periodontal space present between the cementum and the alveolus. The main function of the periodontium is to attach the tooth to the bone. Other important functions include (i) to act as a shock absorber, (ii) to play a role in tooth eruption, and (iii) form and maintain tissues like PDL, cementum, and bone. The role of the PDL during orthodontic tooth movement (OTM) is vital as a healthy PDL facilitates movement by getting compressed on the pressure side and stretched on the tension side. The PDL is widest at the crest area, followed by the apical area. It originates from the dental follicle or sac, just like cementum and alveolar bone. With increasing age, cells, vascularity, and thickness of the PDL decreases and stones called cementicles may

An Illustrated Guide to Oral Histology, First Edition. Edited by Imran Farooq, Saqib Ali, and Paul Anderson.
© 2021 John Wiley & Sons Ltd. Published 2021 by John Wiley & Sons Ltd.
Companion website: www.wiley.com/go/farooq/oral_histology

Table 6.1 Different types and subtypes of principal collagen fibers.

Principal collagen fibers of PDL	Further subtypes
1. Gingival fibers	Dentogingival fibers, alveologingival fibers, circular fibers, dentoperiosteal fibers, transseptal fibers
2. Alveolodental ligament	Alveolar crest fibers, horizontal fibers, oblique fibers, apical fibers, and interradicular fibers

become evident. The two main components of the PDL include cells and fibers. Among its cell population, many essential cells are present including fibroblasts, osteoblasts, cementoblasts, undifferentiated mesenchymal cells, macrophages, lymphocytes, mast cells, and epithelial rest cells. The fibers of the PDL are divided into principal collagen and elastic types. The principal collagen fibers will be discussed later in this chapter. The elastic type includes oxytalan, elaunin, and elastin fibers. Among these, oxytalan fibers are important as they are embedded on one end in bone or cementum and at the other end in smooth muscle associated with blood vessels. Therefore, it is not surprising that they support blood vessels, nerves, and help fibroblast migration. The space between the fibers is filled with interstitial tissue which allows for the vascular and functional needs of the PDL. The principal collagen fibers are divided into two types (Table 6.1).

6.1 Gingival Fibers

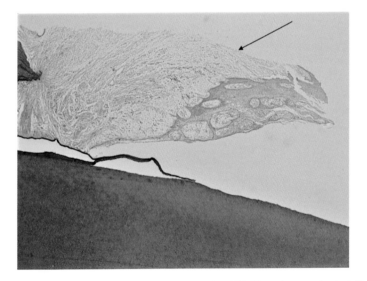

Figure 6.2 H and E stained section showing PDL fibers (arrow, gingival fiber group).

6.1.1 Description

The gingival fibers are principal fibers of the PDL which are present in the gingival area. They consist of five groups (depending on the orientation of the fibers): dentogingival fibers, alveologingival group, circular group, dentoperiosteal group, and transseptal fiber. These fibers are mostly

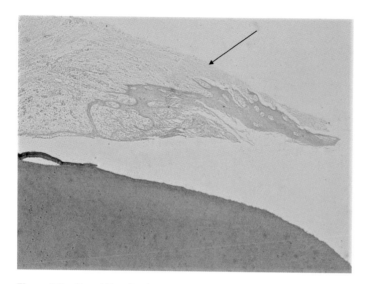

Figure 6.3 H and E stained section showing PDL fibers (arrow, gingival fiber group).

composed of type I collagen although type III collagen could also be found. Unlike most other PDL fibers which are present between teeth and alveolar bone, gingival group fibers attach the tooth with the gingival tissue (except transseptal which is connected between two adjacent teeth). The dentogingival fibers arise from the cementum and extend toward lamina propria of free and attached gingiva. This group of fibers is the most abundant among all gingival fibers. The alveologingival group arises from the crest of the alveolar bone and extends toward the lamina propria of free and attached gingiva. The circular group forms a cuff or circular band around the tooth's neck, inter-winding with corresponding fibers of the same group. These are smaller in number as compared to the others in this group. The dentoperiosteal group after arising from tooth's cementum runs apically over the periosteum and inserts into the alveolar bone or the vestibular muscle and floor of the mouth.

6.1.2 Key Identifying Features

On histological examination, it is difficult to identify individual fibers in this group. However, gingival group as a whole can be easily seen on the side of the tooth, just above alveolar crest of the bone. They cuff around the neck of the tooth like a collar.

6.1.3 Clinical Significance

Gingival fibers tend to support the attachment of gingiva to the tooth's structure [1]. With the application of incisal/occlusal pressure, gingival fibers are consequently stretched indicating the supportive role in attachment [2]. These fibers form the first line of defense against periodontitis as once they are breached, they cannot regenerate and their loss results in accumulation of more plaque and bacteria in gingival sulcus [3].

6.2 Transseptal Fibers

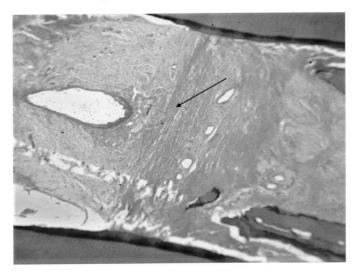

Figure 6.4 H and E stained section showing PDL fibers (arrow, transseptal fiber group).

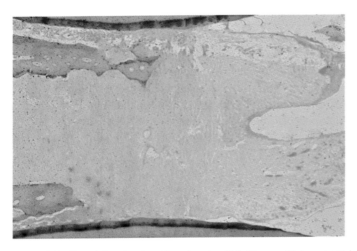

Figure 6.5 H and E stained section showing PDL fibers with transseptal fibers in between the teeth.

6.2.1 Description

Transseptal fibers of the PDL are also known as interdental ligament. Although they are considered part of the gingival fibers (as they do not possess any osseous attachment), they are discussed separately here. These fibers are situated interproximally and extend from the mesial surface cementum of one tooth to the distal surface cementum of the adjacent tooth, except for the central incisors where the fibers arise and insert into the mesial surfaces of the teeth. These fibers possess self-renewal and regeneration capability. They form horizontal collagen bundles just apical to the junctional epithelium and play a role in maintaining structural integrity of the gingiva.

6.2.2 Key Identifying Features

Histologically, they are easily located between the cementum of adjacent teeth. They arise from the cementum of one tooth in the form of bundles and insert into the neighboring tooth's cementum stretching over the interdental bone present between the teeth.

6.2.3 Clinical Significance

Transseptal fibers' primary role is to act as a chain-like structure by holding the teeth together in harmony and synchrony [4]. These fibers collectively form an interdental ligament by connecting all teeth in the arch and appear to be uniquely important in maintaining the integrity of the dental arch [4]. Transseptal fiber system resists tooth separation (mesial and distal) and helps to ensure that teeth remain in proper relationship to one another [1]. During mastication, food is deflected toward the opposing arch by this interdental ligament [5]. These fibers also limit the zone of inflammation by precluding the inflammation from entering the alveolar crest during severe gingivitis [6]. In orthodontically treated patients, a higher incidence of relapse exists in rotated teeth and transseptal fibers are mostly responsible [1]. In these cases, transseptal fibrotomy provides positive stability post-orthodontic treatment [7]. The contraction of transseptal fibers is also thought to play a role in mesial drifting of the dentition [5]. In an animal study, spacing was created between a monkey's teeth and it was observed that teeth moved separately in the absence of transseptal fibers and closer to each other, when transseptal fibers were present [8].

6.3 Alveolar Crest Fibers

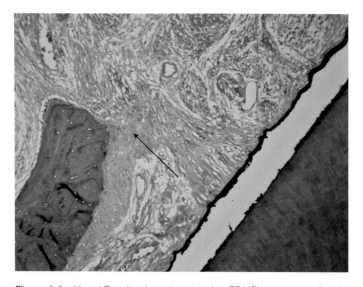

Figure 6.6 H and E stained section showing PDL fibers (arrow, alveolar crest fibers).

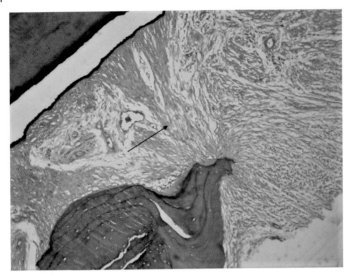

Figure 6.7 H and E stained section showing PDL fibers (arrow, alveolar crest fibers).

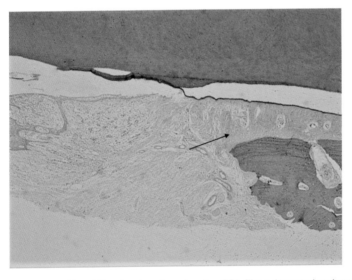

Figure 6.8 H and E stained section showing PDL fibers (arrow, alveolar crest fibers).

6.3.1 Description

Alveolar crest fibers belong to the alveolodental ligament group. They can be found at the location of alveolar crest, arising from the highest point of alveolar bone (margin of bone surrounding the tooth) radiating toward the cementum. Among alveolodental ligament, alveolar crest fibers are furthest away from the apical area of the tooth. In a healthy PDL, all normal cell types like fibroblasts, cementoblasts, epithelial rest cells, undifferentiated mesenchymal cells, and connective tissue cells can be found associated with these fibers. Alveolar crest fibers deliver a load transfer between the tooth and the bone, hence reducing stress on the tooth structure. Like other fibers of the PDL, alveolar crest fibers are viscoelastic, provide cushioning effect during mastication, and play a role in the retention of the tooth in its socket.

6.3.2 Key Identifying Features

As their name indicates, alveolar crest fibers can be seen originating from the crest of the alveolar bone radiating toward the cementum in the cervical area of the tooth. Orientation wise, they are apically inclined with attachment of fibers on the cementum being at a higher level than attachment on the bone.

6.3.3 Clinical Significance

The arrangement of alveolar crest fibers as shown in the Figures 6.6–6.8 enables us to see how they function to resist any lateral forces [5]. This resistance helps retain the tooth in the socket and also protect the deeper fibers present apically [1]. These fibers are also responsible for the prevention of extrusion of teeth particularly related to bending forces during mastication [9]. The alveolar crest fibers first appear obliquely since the crest of the bone is above the CEJ during development [1]. The eruptive tooth movement modifies the initial arrangement of fibers leading to a horizontal direction of fibers followed by its final oblique arrangement after the tooth contacts its counterpart from the opposing arch [1, 4].

6.4 Horizontal Fibers

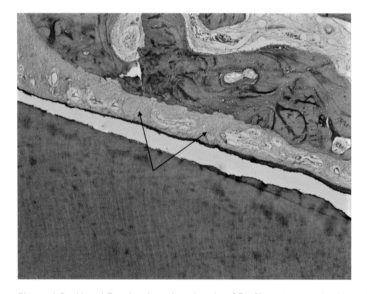

Figure 6.9 H and E stained section showing PDL fibers (arrows, horizontal fibers).

6.4.1 Description

This group of principal fibers is located apical to the alveolar crest fibers group. Horizontal fibers are found near the alveolar crest running at right angles to the long axis of the tooth, connecting its cementum with the bone. Passing from the cemental attachment, these fibers directly cross the periodontal space and insert as Sharpey's fibers.

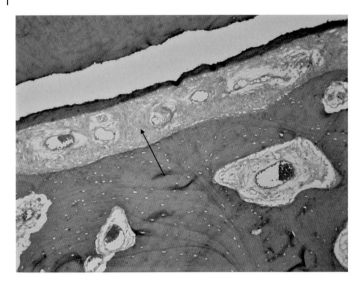

Figure 6.10 H and E stained section showing PDL fibers (arrow, horizontal fibers).

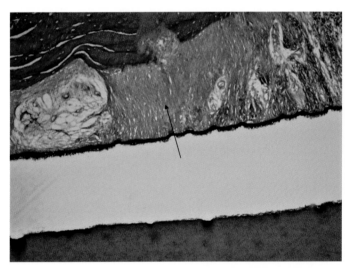

Figure 6.11 H and E stained section showing PDL fibers (arrow, horizontal fibers).

6.4.2 Key Identifying Features

The horizontal fibers group (as shown in the Figures 6.9–6.11) can be seen radiating perpendicularly from the tooth's cementum underneath the crest of the alveolar bone in a horizontal direction. On histological sections, visible attached gingiva with free gingiva present coronally to horizontal fibers can be seen.

6.4.3 Clinical Significance

The orientation of these fiber bundles is relative to their location and therefore, classified accordingly. Horizontal fibers are found below alveolar crest fibers adjacent to the alveolar bone proper and help in resisting horizontal and tipping forces on the tooth [1]. The principal fibers play a key role in tooth eruption and the horizontal fibers along with alveolar crest and dentogingival fibers seem organized upon eruption of succedanous teeth while fibers in the apical region are still in developmental stages [10]. OTM is facilitated by dental tissues and its surrounding structures when exposed to varying degrees of orthodontic force [11]. When the applied forces exceed a threshold, cells of the PDL may die and changes may occur in the orientation of the collagenous periodontal fibers from horizontal to vertical [11].

6.5 Oblique Fibers

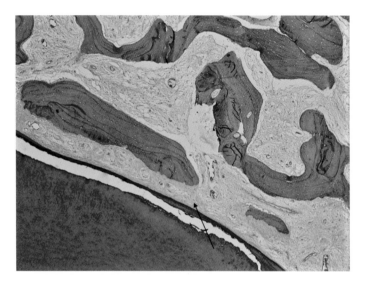

Figure 6.12 H and E stained section showing PDL fibers (arrow, oblique fibers).

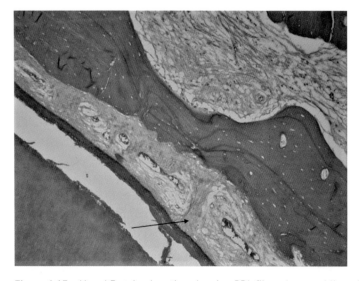

Figure 6.13 H and E stained section showing PDL fibers (arrow, oblique fibers).

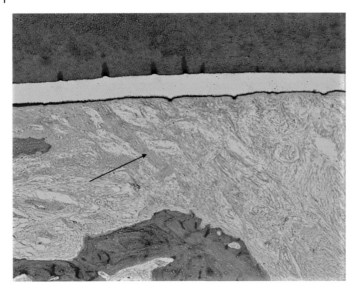

Figure 6.14 H and E stained section showing PDL fibers (arrow, oblique fibers).

6.5.1 Description

This group of fibers of the PDL are present apical to the horizontal fibers. This fiber group is attached obliquely or diagonally to the cementum of the tooth and bone of the tooth socket. They are typically found just above the apical zone of the root adjacent to the alveolar bone. These fibers are the most numerous in number in the PDL and provide the main masticatory support against chewing forces.

6.5.2 Key Identifying Features

These fibers have an oblique orientation with their attachment in the bone at a higher level than the attachment on cementum. This difference in attachment level gives the classic oblique appearance.

6.5.3 Clinical Significance

The function of oblique fibers can be understood by imagining pressure being applied vertically to the incisal (or occlusal) surface of the tooth. Such a pressure will stretch the oblique fibers taut resulting in a pulling rather than a pressure/pushing force on both the cementum and bone of the alveolus (tooth socket) [12]. This pull or tension force is beneficial as continued pressure on bone will result in bone or cementum resorption [12]. These fibers resist vertical and intrusive forces and can absorb significant vertical masticatory pressures and transmit these in the form of tension to the alveolar bone [1].

6.6   Apical Fibers

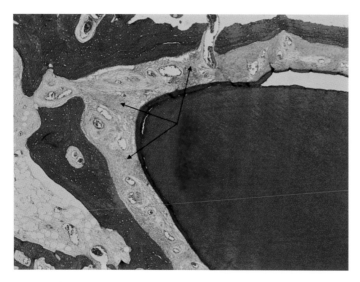

Figure 6.15   H and E stained section showing PDL fibers (arrows, apical fibers).

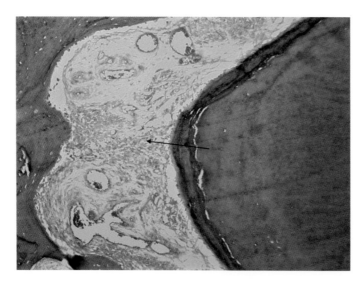

Figure 6.16   H and E stained section showing PDL fibers (arrows, apical fibers).

6.6.1   Description

Apical fibers are so called because of their unique location in the apical area between the cementum of the tooth apex and alveolar bone. They form a soft base for the tooth socket and among alveolodental ligament; these are furthest away from the coronal area of the tooth. These fibers are primarily made up of collagen type I although some type III collagen also exists.

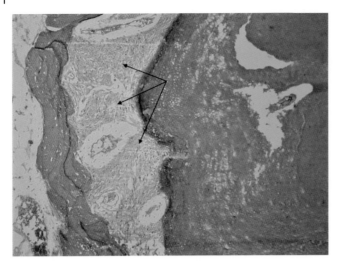

Figure 6.17 H and E stained section showing PDL fibers (arrows, apical fibers).

6.6.2 Key Identifying Features

Apical fibers radiate perpendicular to their attachment from cementum and extend toward the bottom of the fundic alveolar bone. Under high magnification, they have a fine brush-like appearance.

6.6.3 Clinical Significance

These fibers resist apically directed vertical and intrusive forces [1]. The apical fibers also have a key role in the attachment of the tooth in the socket [5]. As root resorption during OTM mostly occurs at the apical area, the role of these fibers becomes very important to allow sufficient movement [13]. Damage of apical fibers particularly due to trauma could lead to ankylosis [14].

6.7 Interradicular Fibers

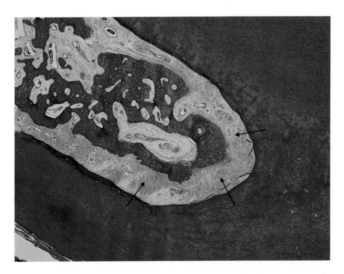

Figure 6.18 H and E stained section showing PDL fibers (arrows, interradicular fibers).

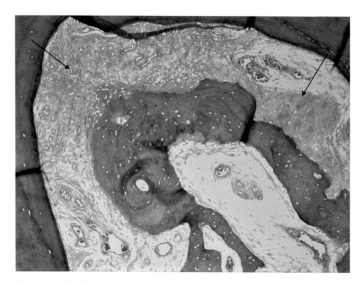

Figure 6.19 H and E stained section showing PDL fibers (arrows, interradicular fibers).

6.7.1 Description

Interradicular fibers are present in between the roots (bifurcation) of multirooted teeth (i.e. premolars and molars). They are attached between the interradicular bone and cementum of the root. These collagenous bundles are approximately 5 μm thick.

6.7.2 Key Identifying Features

These collagen fibers are found in the interradicular/bifurcation area of the tooth present between interradicular bone and cementum of the tooth.

6.7.3 Clinical Significance

The function of interradicular fibers of multirooted teeth is to stabilize the tooth by resisting vertical and lateral movements [5]. Damage of the interradicular region can be related to endodontic causes or plaque accumulation, hence correct diagnosis plays a vital role for correct therapy [15]. When the interradicular region is affected due to periodontitis, the inflammation leads to gingival recession and formation of gingival pockets [16]. The eventual outcome is destruction of both PDL and bone, causing mobility and loss of teeth if the problem persists [16].

6.8 Gingivitis

6.8.1 Description

Gingivitis means inflammation of the gingiva. It has many types and most of its forms are plaque-induced. Plaque is a biofilm that is composed of water, bacteria, polysaccharides, and glycoproteins. Gingivitis may or may not progress into periodontitis but the latter is always preceded by the former. This disease can be reversed by maintaining proper oral hygiene. The signs and symptoms of gingivitis include inflamed and bleeding gingiva (upon brushing and touching); bright red appearance; tender, painful, and swollen gingiva; receding gum line; and halitosis.

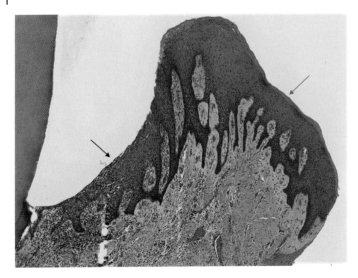

Figure 6.20 H and E stained section showing gingivitis (blue arrow, smooth gingiva; black arrow, sulcular epithelium). Note normal attachment of junctional epithelium and inflammation in the connective tissue.

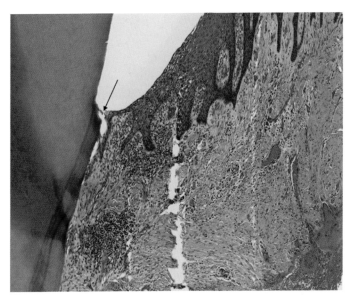

Figure 6.21 H and E stained section showing edematous sulcular and junctional epithelium attached at CEJ with no apical migrations (arrow, junctional epithelial attachment).

6.8.2 Key Identifying Features

Normal gingiva has a textured surface due to the presence of stippling. The stippling or orange-peel look is characteristic of healthy gingiva. On histological sections, gingivitis appears with the smooth gingiva. There is also loss of the normal gingival stippling, inflammation, and widening of the sulcus (leading to false pocket formation).

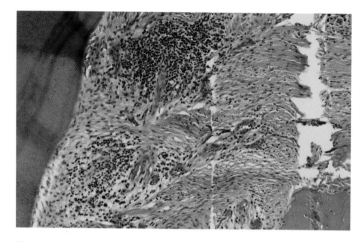

Figure 6.22 High-power H and E stained section of gingivitis showing aggregates of inflammation but no disruption of PDL fibers. The attachments to cementum (left) and bone (right) are also intact.

6.8.3 Clinical Considerations

Bleeding of gingiva is a common sign but there is no gingival recession or bone loss [17]. Gingivitis could be plaque-induced or may be caused by underlying diseases, use of certain medications, malnutrition, trauma, and foreign body reactions [18]. Gingivits could be prevented by flossing daily, in addition to toothbrushing [19]. There is also evidence that the use of rotatory toothbrushes could lead to a higher reduction in gingivitis as compared to manual toothbrushing [20]. Gingivitis could be treated at home by adequately removing plaque through brushing and flossing, although a visit to the dentist to remove plaque and calculus deposits through scaling is mostly advised [17]. Surgical reduction of hyperplastic tissue may be required also. This is carried out by a periodontist through gingivoplasty or gingivectomy [21].

6.9 Periodontitis

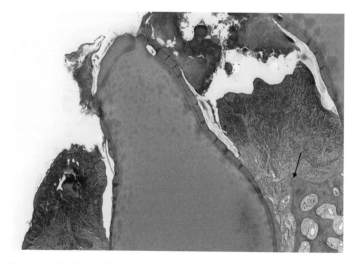

Figure 6.23 H and E stained section showing periodontitis (arrow, loss of alveolar bone with typical notching).

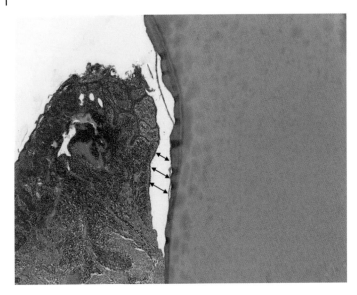

Figure 6.24   H and E stained section showing periodontitis (arrows, gingival detachment and apical migration).

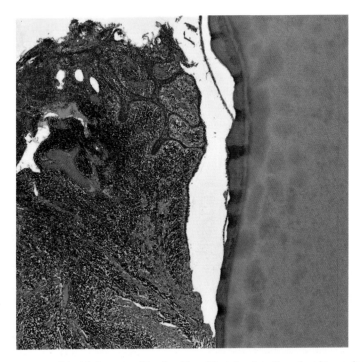

Figure 6.25   Higher magnification H and E stained section showing periodontitis with gingival detachment and apical migration. Note the dense chronic inflammatory aggregates and pocket formation.

6.9.1 Description

Periodontitis is advanced inflammation that results in damage of the supporting bone and soft tissues of teeth. Progression of gingivitis into periodontitis involves detachment and apical migration of junctional epithelium (which lies at the depth of gingival sulcus) to form a pocket. Periodontitis has three major types: necrotizing periodontal diseases, periodontitis as a manifestation of systemic diseases, and periodontitis (based on severity, complexity, extent, and grades). Periodontal regeneration is an important phenomenon but once periodontitis has established, relying only on natural regeneration is not a viable option. The signs and symptoms of periodontitis include red bleeding swollen gingiva, halitosis, gingival recession, deep pockets, and mobile teeth due to the loss of alveolar bone.

6.9.2 Key Identifying Features

Major findings that are easily recognizable on histological sections of periodontitis are detachment of junctional epithelium from the ACJ with apical migration, inflammation, and loss of alveolar bone.

6.9.3 Clinical Considerations

The strategies to prevent periodontitis are similar to that of the prevention of gingivitis, i.e. flossing every day and twice-daily toothbrushing [19]. Treatment of periodontitis is challenging and requires utmost cooperation from the patient as well. Therapeutic interventions include proper maintenance of oral hygiene, cessation of smoking, dietary modifications, and in-office plaque and calculus removal through subgingival instrumentation [22]. Patients are not required to be on antibiotic therapy for the treatment of periodontitis as long as they do not show systemic symptoms [23].

References

1 Nanci, A. and Ten, C.A.R. (2003). *Ten Cate's Oral Histology: Development, Structure, and Function.* St. Louis, MO: Mosby.
2 Jati, A.S., Furquim, L.Z., and Consolaro, A. (2016). Gingival recession: its causes and types, and the importance of orthodontic treatment. *Dental Press J Orthod* 21 (3): 18–29.
3 Itoiz, M.E. and Carranza, F.A. (2002). The gingiva. In: *Carranza's Clinical Periodontology*, 9e (eds. M.G. Newman, H.H. Takei and F.A. Carranza), 26–27. Philadelphia: W.B. Saunders Company.
4 Bathla, S. (2011). *Periodontics Revisited*, 1e. India: Jaypee Brothers Medical Publishers.
5 Berkovitz, B., Holland, G., and Moxham, B. (2017). *Oral Anatomy, Histology and Embryology*, 5e. Elsevier 472 p.
6 Goldman, H.M. (1957). The behavior of transseptal fibres in periodontal disease. *J Dent Res* 36 (2): 249–254.
7 Parker, G.R. (1972). Transseptal fibres and relapse following bodily retration of teeth: a histologic study. *Am J Orthod* 61 (4): 331–344.
8 Moss, J.P. and Picton, D.C. (1982). Short-term changes in the mesiodistal position of teeth following removal of approximal contacts in the monkey Macaca fascicularis. *Arch Oral Biol* 27: 273–278.

9 Popowics, T., Boyd, T., and Hinderberger, H. (2014). Eruptive and functional changes in periodontal ligament fibroblast orientation in CD44 wild-type vs. knockout mice. *J Periodontal Res* 49 (3): 355–362.

10 Beertsen, W., McCulloch, C.A., and Sodek, J. (1997). The periodontal ligament: a unique, multifunctional connective tissue. *Periodontol 2000* 13: 20–40.

11 Maltha, J.C., Vandevska-Radunovic, V., and Kuijpers-Jagtman, A.M. (2015). *The Biological Background of Relapse of Orthodontic Tooth Movement. Biological Mechanisms of Tooth Movement*, 248–259. Chichester: Wiley.

12 Melfi, R.C. and Alley, K.E. (2000). *Permar's Oral Embryology & Microscopic Anatomy*, 10e. LWW.

13 Feller, L., Khammissa, R.A., Thomadakis, G. et al. (2016). Apical external root resorption and repair in orthodontic tooth movement: biological events. *Biomed Res Int* 2016: 4864195.

14 Solanki, G., Lohra, N., and Solanki, R. (2014). The importance of periodontal fibres: a review. *Ind J Pharm Sci Res* 4 (3): 192–193.

15 Carnevale, G., Pontoriero, R., and Hürzeler, M.B. (1995). Management of furcation involvement. *Periodontology 2000* 9 (1): 69–89.

16 Cope, G. and Cope, A. (2011). The periodontium: an anatomical guide. *Dent. Nursing* 7 (7): 376–378.

17 Coventry, J., Griffiths, G., Scully, C., and Tonetti, M. (2000). ABC of oral health: periodontal disease. *BMJ* 321 (7252): 36–39.

18 Caton, J.G., Armitage, G., Berglundh, T. et al. (2018). A new classification scheme for periodontal and peri-implant diseases and conditions: introduction and key changes from the 1999 classification. *J Clin Periodontol* 45 (Suppl 20): S1–S8.

19 Sambunjak, D., Nickerson, J.W., Poklepovic, T. et al. (2011). Flossing for the management of periodontal diseases and dental caries in adults. *Cochrane Database Syst Rev* (12): CD008829.

20 Deacon, S.A., Glenny, A.M., Deery, C. et al. (2010). Different powered toothbrushes for plaque control and gingival health. *Cochrane Database Syst Rev* (12): CD004971.

21 Prichard, J. (1961). Gingivoplasty, gingivectomy, and osseous surgery. *J Periodont* 32 (4): 275–282.

22 Graziani, F., Karapetsa, D., Alonso, B. et al. (2017). Nonsurgical and surgical treatment of periodontitis: how many options for one disease? *Periodontol 2000* 75 (1): 152–188.

23 Kapoor, A., Malhotra, R., Grover, V., and Grover, D. (2012). Systemic antibiotic therapy in periodontics. *Dent Res J (Isfahan)* 9 (5): 505–515.

7

Alveolar Bone

Rizwan Ullah[1], Shehriar Husain[2], Faraz Mohammed[3], and Syed Ali Khurram[4]

[1] *Department of Oral Biology, Sindh Institute of Oral Health Sciences, Jinnah Sindh Medical University, Karachi, Pakistan*
[2] *Department of Dental Materials Science, Sindh Institute of Oral Health Sciences, Jinnah Sindh Medical University, Karachi, Pakistan*
[3] *Department of Biomedical Dental Sciences, College of Dentistry, Imam Abdulrahman Bin Faisal University, Dammam, Saudi Arabia*
[4] *Unit of Oral and Maxillofacial Pathology, School of Clinical Dentistry, University of Sheffield, Sheffield, United Kingdom*

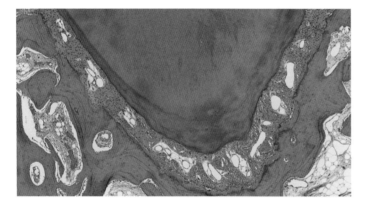

Figure 7.1   H and E stained section showing compact bone outside tooth apex.

The human alveolar bone is very much similar to cementum. It is composed of 67 wt.% inorganic component and 33 wt.% organic material. Inorganic components include hydroxyapatite (HAP) crystals whereas the organic part mostly comprises collagen and a small proportion of protein molecules. The most vital function of alveolar bone is to provide protection to the tooth root, as the blood vessels and nerves enter teeth through the apical foramen. Other functions of alveolar bone include (i) helping in the tooth attachment as periodontal ligament (PDL) fibers insert into it, (ii) serves as a reservoir of minerals, and (iii) proprioception. Bone is formed by cells called osteoblasts and resorbed by osteoclasts whereas osteocytes representing entrapped osteoblasts in the matrix are also easily identified and their presence can be used to determine the vitality of bone. Compared to cementum, bone has a greater remodeling capability. Histologically, two important bone types are compact bone and spongy bone. Compact bone is also called cortical bone whereas the spongy bone has many names such as woven, trabecular, or cancellous bone. Three types of layers (lamellae) are identified in the human alveolar bone which include circumferential, interstitial, and concentric. These

An Illustrated Guide to Oral Histology, First Edition. Edited by Imran Farooq, Saqib Ali, and Paul Anderson.
© 2021 John Wiley & Sons Ltd. Published 2021 by John Wiley & Sons Ltd.
Companion website: www.wiley.com/go/farooq/oral_histology

features, along with other important features and common histological appearance of alveolar bone under normal and certain pathological conditions, are discussed in the following sections.

7.1 Compact Bone

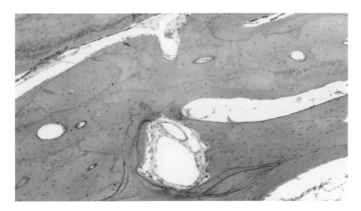

Figure 7.2 H and E stained section of compact bone.

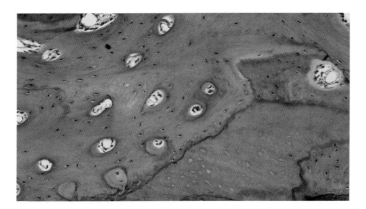

Figure 7.3 H and E stained section of compact bone.

7.1.1 Description

Compact bone forms the outer denser sheet of the alveolar bone. It is also referred to as cortical bone, and cortical means outer shell or cortex. This bone forms a solid dense mass and is covered on the outside by a connective tissue layer called periosteum. The inner surface of connective tissue lining of both compact and spongy bone is called endosteum. Compared to the endosteal surface, periosteal surface is more involved in bone formation. Part of the compact bone which lines the tooth socket is called cribriform plate (resembling a sieve) but on radiographs, it appears as a radiopaque line and is called lamina dura. The thickness of the cribriform plate varies between individuals and is also different for different teeth in the same individual. This bone also forms the buccal and palatal alveolar plates with a considerable amount of spongy bone in between. Strength wise, compact bone boasts stronger and stiffer characteristics when compared with spongy bone. This is mainly due to the lack of marrow or medullary spaces in it.

7.1.2 Key Identifying Features

Compact bone is dense and does not have any hollow spaces or a medullary cavity. The compact bone which lines the tooth socket gives attachment to PDL fibers (alveolodental ligaments), which on the other end are inserted in cementum.

7.1.3 Clinical Significance

The compact bone together with spongy bone forms a system which has superior strength [1]. This arrangement gives it excellent strength, especially against compressive stresses [2]. The main function of compact bone is support and protection of underlying tissues [3].

7.2 Circumferential Lamellae

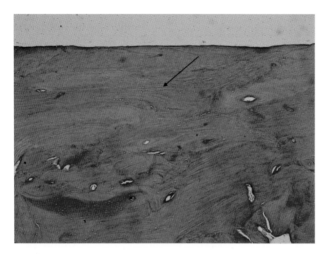

Figure 7.4 H and E stained section of compact bone (arrow, circumferential lamellae).

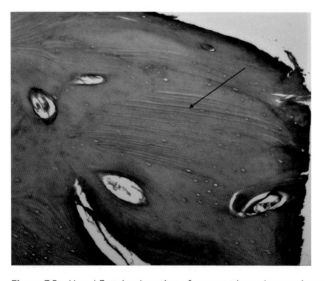

Figure 7.5 H and E stained section of compact bone (arrow, circumferential lamellae).

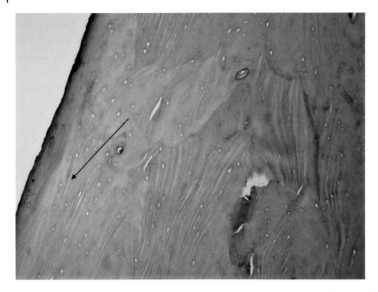

Figure 7.6   H and E stained section of compact bone (arrow, circumferential lamellae).

7.2.1   Description

On the outer and inner circumference or perimeter of compact bone, osteoblasts contribute to the development of lamellae that are called circumferential or longitudinal lamellae. In between these circumferential lamellae (outer and inner circumference of bone), the remaining units of bone are called osteons (i.e. concentric lamellae + haversian canal) and interstitial lamellae. The circumferential lamellae are fewer in number and are arranged either around the wall of the bone marrow (endosteal region) and referred to as inner circumferential lamellae or on the outer border of the bone (periosteal region) and are called outer circumferential lamellae. It should be noted that all compact bone is lamellar and all lamellae contain collagen fibers.

7.2.2   Key Identifying Features

They appear as longitudinal parallel layers of bone which are seen at its outer or inner surface.

7.2.3   Clinical Significance

The inner surface of inner circumferential lamellae comprises bone lining or inactive osteoblasts cells [2]. During bone growth and remodeling, these flat inactive osteoblasts become cuboidal and start synthesizing new un-mineralized lamellar bone called osteoid [3]. This, on mineralization, forms another layer of inner circumferential lamella [4]. A similar process takes place on the outer surface, forming layers of outer circumferential lamellae [4].

7.3 Concentric Lamellae

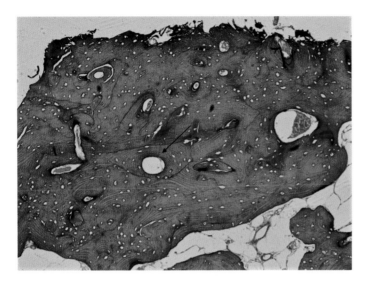

Figure 7.7 H and E stained section of compact bone (arrow, concentric lamellae).

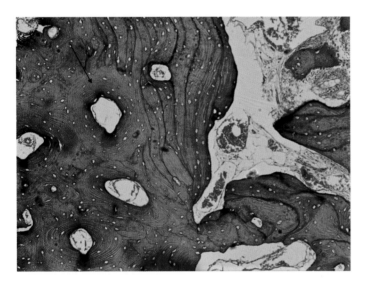

Figure 7.8 H and E stained section of compact bone (arrow, concentric lamellae).

7.3.1 Description

Adult bone is deposited in layers or lamellae. The bulk of compact bone is formed of circular layers known as concentric lamellae. In compact bone, there are lamellae with smaller circular shape (i.e. concentric lamellae) present deeper and associated with a central haversian canal. The thickness of each lamella is approximately 3–5 μm and in the lamellar structure, the collagen and minerals are organized in discrete sheets.

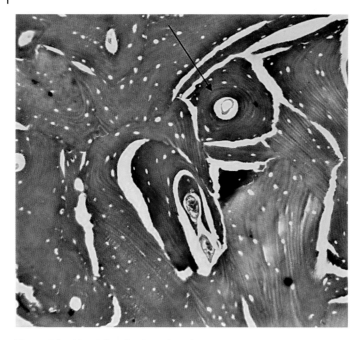

Figure 7.9 H and E stained section of compact bone (arrow, concentric lamellae).

7.3.2 Key Identifying Features

The central neurovascular canal is surrounded by a bone matrix that is concentrically arranged. Microscopically, the concentric lamellae appear like rings in a tree stem. The thin osteocytic lacunae are associated with these lamellae. However, their number depends on the rate of bone formation.

7.3.3 Clinical Significance

The inner surface of concentric lamellae is associated with inactive osteoblasts and when activated, these cells begin forming new lamellar osteoid [4]. This process is prominent during active bone growth. Moreover, it occurs regularly as part of the mechanism responsible for the dynamic refashioning of bone [1].

7.4 Interstitial Lamellae

7.4.1 Description

Interstitial lamellae occupy the space between adjacent concentric lamellae. The interstitial lamellae develop from the remnants of osteons that get incompletely resorbed during bone remodeling. The interstitial lamellae do not have a particular or preferred orientation as they are a consequence of bony remodeling of the haversian system. Their number is higher in the periosteal region compared to endosteal region.

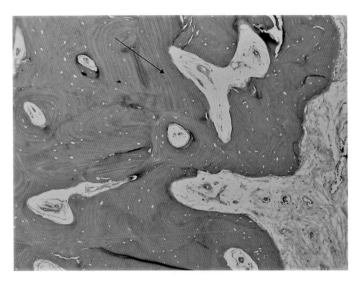

Figure 7.10   H and E stained section of compact bone (arrow, interstitial lamellae).

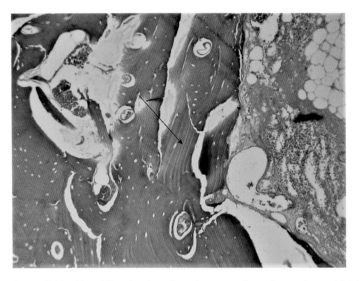

Figure 7.11   H and E stained section of compact bone (arrow, interstitial lamellae).

7.4.2   Key Identifying Features

The interstitial lamellae are present between different concentric lamellae. They do not possess any specific shape as these are residual fragments of osteons.

7.4.3   Clinical Significance

They have no specific clinical significance as they are the residual fragments between the haversian system. However, it was suggested by Goodwin and Sharkey that mechanical properties of the bone are dependent on these lamellae of bone [5].

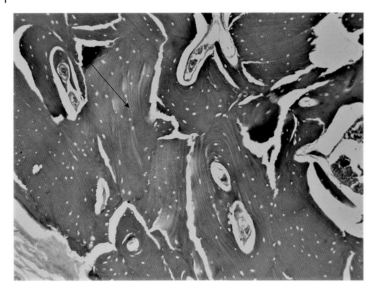

Figure 7.12 H and E stained section of compact bone (arrow, interstitial lamellae).

7.5 Osteocytes and Lacunae

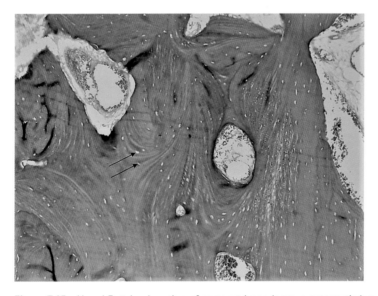

Figure 7.13 H and E stained section of compact bone (arrows, osteocytic lacunae).

7.5.1 Description

In living bone, osteocytic lacunae contain osteocytes and they are the most abundant cells within the bone. These cells make up around 90–95% of all the bone cells. In the matrix of bone, the osteocytes are known to survive for decades. Osteocytes are best described as inactive osteoblasts trapped within the bone matrix during bone formation. The osteocytes, together with the osteoblasts and bone lining cells, are derived from mesenchymal or ectomesenchymal stem cells. The osteocytic lacunae or spaces are dispersed throughout the bone matrix. When bone is rapidly formed (such as during embryonic bone formation and fracture repair), the osteocytic lacunae are large and irregularly spaced. On the other hand, in slowly forming bone, the osteocytic lacunae are small in diameter and are distributed at regular intervals within the matrix of bone.

7.5.2 Key Identifying Features

The lacunae appear as small spaces within the bone matrix that are filled with cell debris or air. These spaces are regularly distributed throughout the bone matrix with no preferential orientation. The number of these spaces varies according to the site and age of bone. Majority of the osteocytic lacunae are present at the interface of the incremental lines, indicating the presence of an interface between new and old bone.

7.5.3 Clinical Significance

The osteocytic lacunae have associated dendritic processes and their role is to help in providing nutrition to the bone through diffusion of nutrients throughout the bone matrix which is essential for maintaining viability [6]. Osteocytes present within the osteocytic lacunae also play an important role in bony remodeling as they are responsible for sending appropriate signals under mechanical straining which can result in the formation or resorption of bone [7]. In addition to maintaining the bone matrix, osteocytes play an important role in osteoclast activation through numerous mechanisms including the expression of receptor activator of nuclear factor kappa-B ligand (RANKL) gene [8]. The osteocytes are considered to be good sensors of biochemical changes in the adjacent environment which helps in homeostasis of calcium in the body [9]. Osteocytes mediate the deposition and release of calcium within bone matrix and therefore, osteocytes present within osteocytic lacunae play a substantial role in maintaining integrity of bone [10].

7.6 Haversian Canals

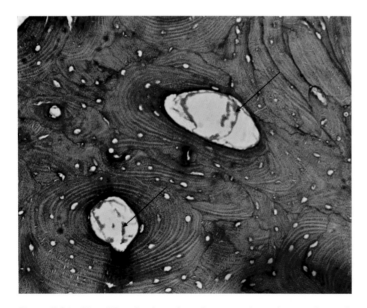

Figure 7.14 H and E stained section of compact bone (arrows, haversian canals).

7.6.1 Description

In the center of concentric lamellae, a central canal is present. This canal is known as the "haversian" or "osteonal" canal. Haversian canals are a series of microscopic tubes that appear as large, circular, or oval spaces with an approximate diameter of 50 μm.

7.6.2 Key Identifying Features

Usually in histological sections, these canals appear empty but occasionally these canals contain remnants of blood vessel endothelium and blood cells. In the longitudinal sections, these haversian canals are interconnected with each other through canals known as Volkmann's canals.

7.6.3 Clinical Significance

The haversian canals in living bone contain blood vessels, nerves, and lymphatics [11]. This profuse and intricate network of blood and nerve serves to nourish, sustain, and provide sensory supply to bone [12]. Therefore, sometimes these haversian canals are also referred to as nutrient canals [11]. The surfaces of the haversian canals also act as sites for bone deposition and bone resorption and this is due to the presence of bone cells lining the haversian canal's inner perimeter [1]. Water is among one of the important constituents of bone constituting about 10–20% of the total bone volume and one important location that holds this water component is the haversian canal (other locations for water compartment include bone marrow, canaliculi, inside collagen fibers, interface of collagen-mineral, and within crystal lattice) [13]. This water compartment has a profound impact on the mechanical properties of bone and also aids the process of metabolites exchange and ion transport between the cells and within different regions of bone [14]. The number of haversian canals present in a region changes throughout life and increasing numbers are seen with growing age which may assist in human age estimation [15].

7.7 Volkmann's Canals

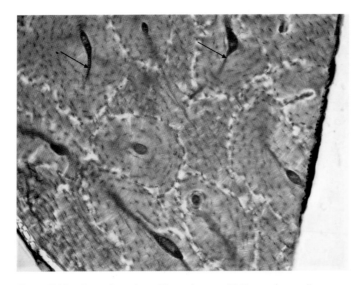

Figure 7.15 Ground section of bone (arrows, Volkmann's canal).

7.7.1 Description

Volkmann's canals are located perpendicular to the haversian canals. They are responsible for forming a network with the haversian canal, medullary cavity, and with the outer bone surface. These canals are also referred to as transverse perforating canals. They contain the same neuro-vascular bundles that are present in the haversian canal.

7.7.2 Key Identifying Features

These canals extend in various directions at random angles. In cross sections of bone, the Volkmann's canals are partially visible. In the longitudinal sections, complete Volkmann's canals are visible connecting the adjacent haversian canals, with the medullary cavity and with the peri-osteum of the bone forming a complete interconnecting network.

7.7.3 Clinical Significance

Volkmann's canals connect the periosteal blood and nerve vessels to the central supply [11]. They form an intricate network via anastomoses with the adjacent nerve and blood vessels [16]. This in turn contributes to the rich blood and nerve supply of bone, building a strong communication network between the adjacent osteons and also between the endosteal and periosteal bone surfaces [17]. There are higher number of Volkmann's canals in the alveolar bone due to requirement of profuse blood supply to the PDL cells and due to the presence of these canals, the alveolar bone has a "sieve"-like appearance [1]. The bone in the alveolar socket is therefore commonly referred to as cribriform plate [18].

7.8 Osteons

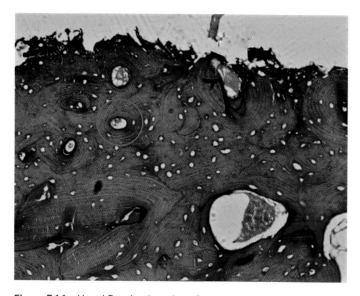

Figure 7.16 H and E stained section of compact bone (green circle, osteon).

7.8.1 Description

The osteon is another term used for referring to the haversian system, comprising the haversian canal and concentric lamellae. The osteons form the most important structural unit of compact bone and are further classified into primary and secondary osteons. The primary osteons have a diameter of 50–100 μm with a few lamellae (<10 in number). The secondary osteons on the other hand are larger in diameter (100–250 μm) and have a greater number of concentric lamellae (20–25 in number) [9]. Their usual orientation is parallel to the long axis of the bone. The size and number of osteons varies with age and they become more numerous but smaller with increasing age.

7.8.2 Key Identifying Features

The haversian system or osteon consists of concentric layers organized around a central neurovascular canal known as haversian canal. The central canal comprises blood vessel, nerves, and lymphatics in living bone. Each osteon is bounded by a prominent incremental line rich in collagen that demarcates the osteon from the rest of interstitial bone.

7.8.3 Clinical Significance

The osteon is an integral structural and functional unit within the bone architecture [19]. In light of this, the weight bearing role is crucial for buttressing against bending and torsional forces [12]. Osteons are organized along the stress lines and this arrangement helps the bone to resist fractures [1].

7.9 Spongy Bone

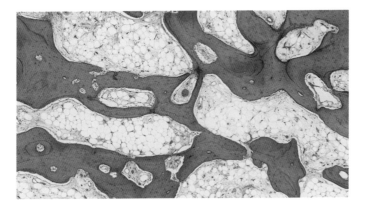

Figure 7.17 H and E stained section of spongy bone showing bony trabeculae.

7.9.1 Description

Spongy bone (also called cancellous bone or trabecular bone) consists of a network of fine, irregular bony plates called trabeculae which are separated by interconnecting spaces. It forms around 15% of the bony skeleton while the remaining 85% is formed by the compact bone. The thickest trabeculae are usually seen in the alveolar bone compared to other sites in the body where trabeculae are fine and thin.

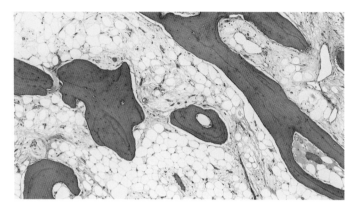

Figure 7.18 H and E stained section of spongy bone showing bony trabeculae.

7.9.2 Key Identifying Features

Bony trabeculae are irregular in shape and are found at spaces from each other. In between bony trabeculae, there are fibrofatty marrow spaces. As the histological structure resembles a sponge, this bone is called spongy bone.

7.9.3 Clinical Significance

The primary function of trabecular bone is mineral metabolism and thus it has a higher turnover rate compared to compact bone [20]. The bone is not spongy from the mechanical point of view as it has specialized orientation of trabeculae in long bones that can distribute the loads, rather it is called spongy or trabecular bone because of its structure and organization [1]. The mechanical and protective roles are secondary functions of trabecular bone [14]. These trabeculae are not random in orientation within bone and the patterns formed are a visual manifestation of the lines of stress, reflecting the forces acting on the structure of bone and its inherent ability to withstand them [21].

7.10 Marrow Spaces

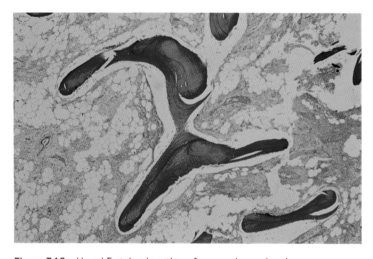

Figure 7.19 H and E stained section of spongy bone showing marrow spaces between trabeculae.

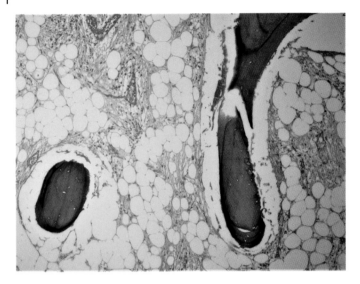

Figure 7.20 H and E stained section of spongy bone showing marrow spaces between trabeculae.

7.10.1 Description

In young bone, the marrow is red and hemopoietic as it is actively forming blood cells. In older bone, these marrow spaces are filled with yellow marrow, as there is loss of hemopoietic potential and accumulation of fat cells within these spaces.

7.10.2 Key Identifying Features

There are macroscopic marrow spaces present in between the fine interconnecting network of bony trabeculae. In the marrow spaces, there are adipocytes (fat cells) that indicate yellow or fatty marrow.

7.10.3 Clinical Significance

The bony trabeculae receive nutrition from the vascular marrow space through the process of diffusion [22]. In younger individuals, these marrow spaces are filled with red marrow which helps in the formation of blood cells [23]. Additionally, these marrow spaces also contain pluripotent stem cells which may differentiate into different cells such as fibroblasts, osteoblasts, adipocytes, chondrocytes, and myoblasts [1].

7.11 Osteoporosis

7.11.1 Description

Osteoporosis is a condition involving calcium loss from bones that contributes toward the formation of thin porous bone. It is a skeletal condition characterized by low bone mass and an increased fragility due to the micro-architectural deficiency of bone tissue. The clinical

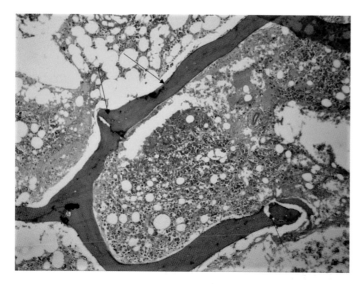

Figure 7.21 H and E stained sections showing osteoporosis (arrows, generalized thinning and irregular trabeculae perforation).

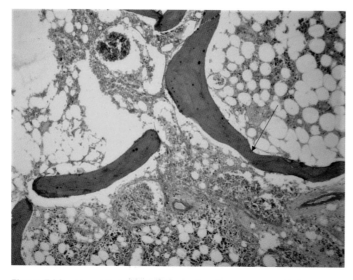

Figure 7.22 H and E stained sections showing osteoporosis (arrow, generalized thinning and irregular trabeculae perforation).

description of osteoporosis is also based on an evaluation of bone mineral density (BMD). As a result of aging, the bone cells begin to remove the matrix of the bone (resorption), while fresh bone cells deposit osteoid formation. This mechanism is called bone remodeling. Bone loss in people with osteoporosis outpaces new bone growth leaving the bones fragile, brittle, and fracture prone. This was once considered a hormonal phenomenon associated with women's aging. Osteoporosis has many causes, including genetic conditions, hormonal problems, and nutritional abnormalities.

7.11.2 Key Identifying Features

The histopathological H and E stained sections in Figures 7.21 and 7.22 show generalized thinning and irregular trabeculae perforation, indicating unbalanced bone resorption induced by osteoclasts. There are large marrow spaces and a thin cortex can also be seen.

7.11.3 Clinical Considerations

Osteoporosis usually occurs in patients who are suffering from other systemic problems [24]. Osteoporosis can occur at any age and is usually associated with diseases that affect calcium and Vitamin D metabolism [25]. Since the bones are thin, they are very prone to fractures [26]. The oral health of these patients is often impaired because of polypharmacy, and due to physical disabilities and insufficient compliance with hygiene guidelines [27]. Preserving the natural dentition of these patients not only is aesthetically pleasing, but also ensures proper intake of balanced nutrition [28].

7.12 Osteomyelitis

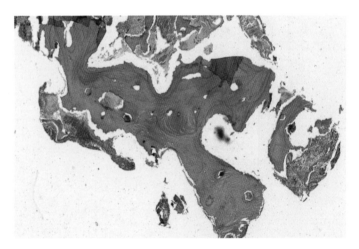

Figure 7.23 H and E stained section showing necrotic bone and depletion of osteocytes from the lacunae seen in osteomyelitis.

7.12.1 Description

The term osteomyelitis can be broken down into "osteo," which means bone, and "myelitis," which means inflammation of the bone's fatty tissues. Osteomyelitis is caused by bone or joint inflammation, which can be further divided into acute and chronic osteomyelitis. It can occur at any age and can involve any bone. Such infections could have bacterial or fungal origin. Osteomyelitis may be caused by trauma, surgery, joint replacement, and/or some form of prosthesis. Acute osteomyelitis is a serious inflammation of the bone which may result from a previous wound, a puncture injury, surgery, bone fracture, tooth abscess, or soft tissue infections. Early diagnosis is very important as timely delivery of antibiotics will prevent irreversible bone loss.

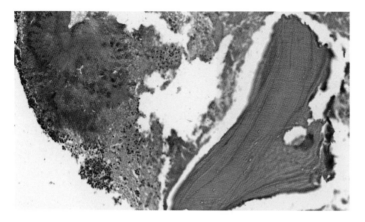

Figure 7.24 H and E stained section showing necrotic bone, depletion of osteocytes from the lacunae, peripheral resorption, and colonization of bacteria seen in osteomyelitis.

7.12.2 Key Identifying Features

The H and E stained parts of histopathologic tissues usually reveal necrotic bone which is identified as sequestrum. The bone reveals the depletion of osteocytes from the lacunae, peripheral resorption, and colonization of bacteria. Acute inflammatory accumulation in haversian canals and peripheral bone comprising polymorphonuclear leukocytes (neutrophils) is also evident.

7.12.3 Clinical Considerations

Most patients with osteomyelitis have symptoms for <2 weeks before being brought to medical attention, although a small proportion also have a low-grade fever and several weeks of sporadic bone pain [29, 30]. The most prevalent symptoms are fever, infection site discomfort, and inability to use an affected extremity [31]. Physical symptoms include a focal swelling, tenderness, warmth, and erythema (usually over a long bone metaphysis) and rarely a draining fistulous tract may develop [29]. Early and effective antibiotic treatment provides the best outcome in patients with osteomyelitis before severe bone loss occurs [32]. Patients should be closely monitored during recovery, for signs and symptoms of worsening infection [32].

7.13 Osteoma

7.13.1 Description

Osteoma is a benign and asymptomatic bone neoplasm, comprising well-differentiated mature tissue. It is distinguished by the multiplication of either compact or cancellous bone at an endosteal or periosteal site. Central osteomas arise from the endosteum whereas peripheral osteomas originate from the periosteum. In terms of pathogenesis, an osteoma could develop as a reaction to trauma, developmental or embryological anomaly, or an inflammatory condition. In many cases, patients are unable to recall a history of trauma. It has also been suggested that chronic infection involving paranasal sinuses can lead to the proliferation of osteogenic cells. The embryological theory suggests that osteomas could originate from the sutures present between bones with

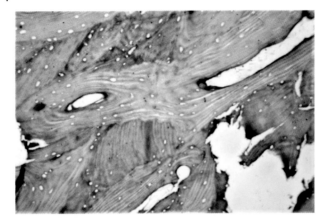

Figure 7.25 H and E stained section of compact osteoma showing mature lamellar bone with absence of haversian canals and fibrous component.

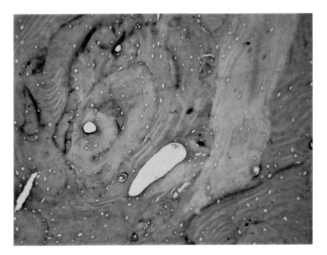

Figure 7.26 H and E stained section of compact osteoma showing mature lamellar bone with absence of haversian canals and fibrous component.

various embryological derivations (endochondral/membranous); however, this is unlikely because osteomas mostly occur in adults (with fused sutures) and not in children.

7.13.2 Key Identifying Features

Decalcified histopathological sections stained with H and E show a compact osteoma comprising mature lamellar bone. There are no haversian canals and no fibrous component. Trabecular osteomas are composed of cancellous trabecular bone with hematopoietic elements surrounded by a cortical bone margin.

7.13.3 Clinical Considerations

The most common symptom of osteoid osteoma is pain [33]. Clinically, osteomas are smaller (10–40 mm) in size; however, if left untreated, they can grow to a larger size and are then called as gigantiform or huge osteomas [34]. With larger lesions, the patient may present with complaints of facial deformity and occlusal dysfunction [35]. The most common presentation are palatal and lingual tori and buccal exostosis.

7.14 Osteitis Deformans (Paget's Disease)

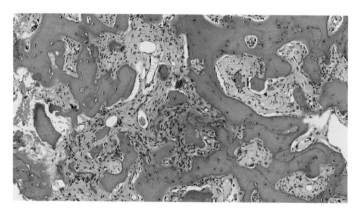

Figure 7.27 H and E stained section showing Paget's disease with chaotic trabeculae (mosaic pattern).

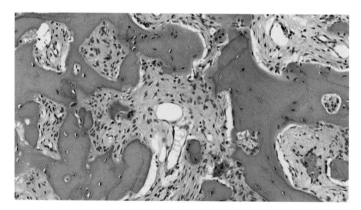

Figure 7.28 H and E stained section of Paget's disease with jigsaw puzzle-like bone (mosaic pattern) and multinucleated osteoclasts.

7.14.1 Description

Paget's disease is also called osteitis deformans. It is a common chronic condition characterized by uncoordinated resorption and deposition of the bone producing large amounts of weak bone. This disease's etiology is unclear, but inflammatory, genetic, and endocrine factors may contribute to this disorder. The pathogenesis of osteitis deformans is described in three stages which are: stage 1: the increase of osteoclastic activity that results in bone degradation; stage 2: in some areas of the bone, both osteoclasts and osteoblasts become overactive, and the rate at which the bone is broken down and reconstructed, increases enormously in the affected areas; and stage 3: in which both osteoclastic and osteoblastic activity ceases, and the bone becomes sclerotic, brittle, and frail.

7.14.2 Key Identifying Features

The histopathological H and E stained sections typically show abnormally large, bizarre osteoclasts. There would be thickened trabeculae, with osteoblasts rimmed on the bone, and stromal cells replacing the marrow. The hallmark mosaic pattern shows randomly arranged lamellar bone segments, with irregular reversal lines. The disarranged woven bone elevates the volume of the bone.

7.14.3 Clinical Considerations

The involvement of jawbone in Paget's disease results in progressive enlargement of bone causing facial asymmetry and pain [36]. A common finding in Paget's disease is hypercementosis which makes dental extractions quite challenging [37]. The bone is highly vascular with numerous arteriovenous shunts during the active disease phase and oral surgical procedures during this phase can lead to severe hemorrhage [38]. The bone is hypersensitive to inflammation during the sclerotic phase and can develop osteomyelitis, even with minimal provocation [38].

7.15 Osteosarcoma

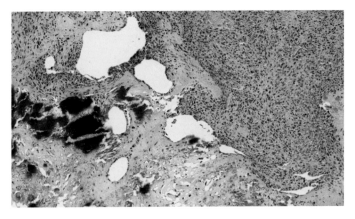

Figure 7.29 H and E stained section of osteosarcoma showing bone fragments on the left, osteoid in the middle, and malignant spindle cells on the right.

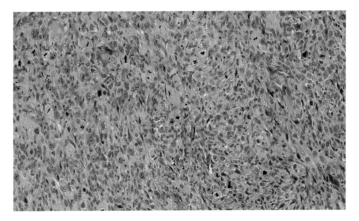

Figure 7.30 H and E stained section of osteosarcoma showing malignant tumor cells with nuclear and cellular pleomorphism, hyperchromatism, and abnormal mitosis.

7.15.1 Description

Osteosarcoma is the most common primary malignant bone tumor. There are numerous variants of osteosarcoma of jawbones, but these are generally classified into two types, i.e. primary and secondary. Osteosarcoma more frequently involves the body's long bones, such as the femur (thigh bone), the tibia (shinbone), or the humerus (bone extending from shoulder to elbow). While they can occur in any bones of the body, jaw tumors only accounts for 7% of all osteosarcomas. Many people diagnosed with osteosarcomas are young (<25 years of age) and males.

7.15.2 Key Identifying Features

The histopathological diagnosis of osteosarcoma is based on recognition of development of abnormal osteoid. Another characteristic microscopic feature is the proliferation of atypical osteoblasts. These cells are arranged in a disorderly fashion and show considerable pleomorphism and hyperchromatism.

7.15.3 Clinical Considerations

Osteosarcomas are classified histopathologically into osteoblastic, chondroblastic, and fibroblastic subtypes. This is determined by the predominant form of extracellular matrix present [39]. Most patients with osteosarcoma have symptoms of persistent pain, swelling, or a firm lump on a bone [40]. Loosening of teeth and paresthesia of the mental nerve are the common manifestations in jaw bones and spontaneous bone fractures may also be seen [41].

References

1 Berkovitz, B.K.B., Holland, G.R., and Moxham, B.J. (2009). *Oral Anatomy, Histology and Embryology*. Edinburgh: Mosby/Elsevier.

2 Nanci, A. and Ten, C.A.R. (2003). *Ten Cate's Oral Histology: Development, Structure, and Function*. St. Louis, MO: Mosby.

3 Florencio-Silva, R., Sasso, G.R., Sasso-Cerri, E. et al. (2015). Biology of bone tissue: structure, function, and factors that influence bone cells. *Biomed Res Int* 421746: 2015.

4 Young, Barbara (Pathologist) (2000). *Wheater's Functional Histology: A Text and Colour Atlas*. Edinburgh; New York: Churchill Livingstone.

5 Goodwin, K.J. and Sharkey, N.A. (2002). Material properties of interstitial lamellae reflect local strain environments. *J Orthop Res* 20 (3): 600–606.

6 Dallas, S.L., Prideaux, M., and Bonewald, L.F. (2013). The osteocyte: an endocrine cell ... and more. *Endocr Rev* 34 (5): 658–690.

7 Bonewald, L.F. and Johnson, M.L. (2008). Osteocytes, mechanosensing and Wnt signaling. *Bone* 42 (4): 606–615.

8 O'Brien, C.A., Nakashima, T., and Takayanagi, H. (2013). Osteocyte control of osteoclastogenesis. *Bone* 54 (2): 258–263.

9 Schaffler, M.B., Cheung, W.Y., Majeska, R., and Kennedy, O. (2014). Osteocytes: master orchestrators of bone. *Calcif Tissue Int* 94 (1): 5–24.

10 Intemann, J., DJJ, D.G., Naylor, A.J. et al. (2020). Importance of osteocyte-mediated regulation of bone remodelling in inflammatory bone disease. *Swiss Med Wkly* 150: w20187.

11 Cowin, S.C. and Cardoso, L. (2015). Blood and interstitial flow in the hierarchical pore space architecture of bone tissue. *J Biomech* 48 (5): 842–854.

12 Bartold, M., Gronthos, S., Haynes, D., and Ivanovski, S. (2019). Mesenchymal stem cells and biologic factors leading to bone formation. *J Clin Periodontol* 46 (Suppl 21): 12–32.

13 Granke, M., Does, M.D., and Nyman, J.S. (2015). The role of water compartments in the material properties of cortical bone. *Calcif Tissue Int* 97 (3): 292–307.

14 Burr, D.B. (2019). *Bone Morphology and Organization. Basic and Applied Bone Biology*, 3–26. Elsevier.

15 Khan, I., Jamil, M.M.A., Ibrahim, T.N.T., and Nor, F.M. (2017). Analysis of age-related changes in Haversian canal using image processing techniques. *Proceedings 6th IEEE International Conference on Control System, Computing and Engineering, ICCSCE 2016*, Penang, Malaysia (25–27 November 2016), 169–172.

16 Marrella, A., Lee, T.Y., Lee, D.H. et al. (2018). Engineering vascularized and innervated bone biomaterials for improved skeletal tissue regeneration. *Mater Today (Kidlington)* 21 (4): 362–376.

17 Chappard, D., Baslé, M.F., Legrand, E., and Audran, M. (2011). New laboratory tools in the assessment of bone quality. *Osteoporos Int* 22 (8): 2225–2240.

18 Mishra, N., Shrivardhan, K., Raviraj, J. et al. (2017). Significance of lamina dura: a review. *Int J Contemp Med Surg Rad* 2 (1): 1–4.

19 Ascenzi, M.G. and Roe, A.K. (2012). The osteon: the micromechanical unit of compact bone. *Front Biosci (Landmark Ed)* 17: 1551–1581.

20 Iolascon, G., Napolano, R., Gioia, M. et al. (2013). The contribution of cortical and trabecular tissues to bone strength: insights from denosumab studies. *Clin Cases Miner Bone Metab* 10 (1): 47–51.

21 Osterhoff, G., Morgan, E.F., Shefelbine, S.J. et al. (2016). Bone mechanical properties and changes with osteoporosis. *Injury* 47 (Suppl 2(Suppl 2)): S11–S20.

22 Zahm, A.M., Bucaro, M.A., Ayyaswamy, P.S. et al. (2010). Numerical modeling of oxygen distributions in cortical and cancellous bone: oxygen availability governs osteonal and trabecular dimensions. *Am J Physiol Cell Physiol* 299 (5): C922–C929.

23 Travlos, G.S. (2006). Histopathology of bone marrow. *Toxicol Path* 34: 566–598.

24 Sözen, T., Özışık, L., and Başaran, N.Ç. (2017). An overview and management of osteoporosis. *Eur J Rheumatol* 4 (1): 46–56.

25 Gourlay, M.L. and Brown, S.A. (2004). Clinical considerations in premenopausal osteoporosis. *Arch Intern Med* 164 (6): 603–614.

26 Warriner, A.H., Patkar, N.M., Curtis, J.R. et al. (2011). Which fractures are most attributable to osteoporosis? *J Clin Epidemiol* 64 (1): 46–53.

27 Kyrgidis, A., Tzellos, T.G., Toulis, K., and Antoniades, K. (2011). The facial skeleton in patients with osteoporosis: a field for disease signs and treatment complications. *J Osteoporos* 2011: 147689.

28 Christensen, L., Hede, B., and Petersen, P. (2005). Public dental health care program for persons with disability. *Acta Odontol Scand* 63 (5): 278–283.

29 Barrett, A.M., Lucero, M.A., Le, T. et al. (2007). Epidemiology, public health burden, and treatment of diabetic peripheral neuropathic pain: a review. *Pain Med* 8 (Suppl 2): S50–S62.

30 Scott, R.J., Christofersen, M.R., Robertson, W.W. et al. (2014). Acute osteomyelitis in children. *N Engl J Med* 370: 352–360.

31 Faden, H. and Grossi, M. (1991). Acute osteomyelitis in children: reassessment of etiologic agents and their clinical characteristics. *Am J Dis Child* 145: 65.

32 Calhoun, J.H., Manring, M.M., and Shirtliff, M. (2009). Osteomyelitis of the long bones. *Semin Plast Surg* 23 (2): 59–72.

33 Noordin, S., Allana, S., Hilal, K. et al. (2018). Osteoid osteoma: contemporary management. *Orthop Rev (Pavia)* 10 (3): 7496.

34 Kaya, G.S., Omezli, M.M., Sipal, S., and Ertas, U. (2010). Oral myiasis: gigantic peripheral osteoma of the mandible. A case report. *J Clin Exp Dent* 2: e160–e162.

35 Kaplan, I., Nicolaou, Z., Hatuel, D., and Calderon, S. (2008). Solitary central osteoma of the jaws: a diagnostic dilemma. *Oral Surg Oral Med Oral Pathol Oral Radiol Endod* 106: e22–e29.

36 Ralston, S.H. (2008). Juvenile Paget's disease, familial expansile osteolysis and other genetic osteolytic disorders. *Best Pract Res Clin Rheumatol* 22: 101–111.

37 Shankar, Y.U., Misra, S.R., Vineet, D.A., and Baskaran, P. (2013). Paget disease of bone: a classic case report. *Contemp Clin Dent* 4 (2): 227–230.

38 Burket, L.W., Greenberg, M.S., and Glick, M. (2003). *Burket's Oral Medicine: Diagnosis & Treatment*. Hamilton, ON: BC Decker.

39 Frei, C., Bornstein, M.M., Stauffer, E. et al. (2004). Osteosarcoma of the maxilla and the maxillary sinus: a case report. *Quintessence Int* 35: 228–233.

40 Arinima, P. and Ishak, A. (2018). Persistent shoulder pain in young male: osteosarcoma. *Korean J Fam Med* 39 (4): 266–269.

41 Slootweg, P.J. and Müller, H. (1985). Osteosarcoma of the jaw bones. Analysis of 18 cases. *J Maxillofac Surg* 13 (4): 158–166.

8

Oral Mucosa

Saqib Ali, Imran Farooq, and Faraz Mohammed

Department of Biomedical Dental Sciences, College of Dentistry, Imam Abdulrahman Bin Faisal University, Dammam, Saudi Arabia

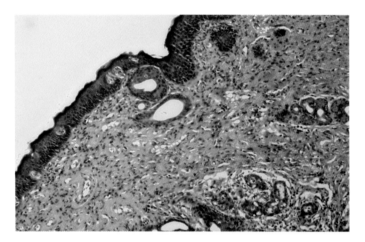

Figure 8.1   H and E stained section showing oral mucosa (mucous membrane of cheek).

Any part of the human body that communicates with the external environment is covered by a moist lining called mucous membrane. In the oral cavity, this membrane is called oral mucosa. Since it is located between skin and pharynx, just like them the oral mucosa has two layers: an outer epithelium and an underlying connective tissue. After the connective tissue, lies submucosa, periosteum, and then the bone. The oral mucosa performs different functions like protection of deeper tissues, sensation of different stimuli, and secretion of saliva. The epithelium of oral cavity is of stratified squamous type and is divided into three major types based on the absence and presence of keratinization: orthokeratinized, parakeratinized, and non-keratinized. Mucosa of the dorsum of the tongue contains four distinct groups of papillae i.e. fungiform, filiform, circumvallate, and foliate papillae (uncommon in humans). Some of these papillae have a mechanical function whereas some contain taste buds and have a function related to taste. The epithelium of fungiform papillae could be keratinized slightly or non-keratinized whereas the epithelium of filiform papillae is always keratinized.

An Illustrated Guide to Oral Histology, First Edition. Edited by Imran Farooq, Saqib Ali, and Paul Anderson.
© 2021 John Wiley & Sons Ltd. Published 2021 by John Wiley & Sons Ltd.
Companion website: www.wiley.com/go/farooq/oral_histology

Although it shows a lot of variations, oral mucosa of humans is mainly divided into masticatory mucosa, lining mucosa, and specialized mucosa. The different types of oral mucosa along with their respective locations are summarized in Table 8.1.

Table 8.1 Showing different types of oral mucosa and their respective location in the oral cavity.

Type of oral mucosa	Location
1. Lining mucosa	Buccal and labial mucosa, alveolar mucosa, floor of the mouth, ventral tongue surface, soft palate, lips (vermillion and intermediate zone)
2. Masticatory mucosa	Attached gingiva, hard palate
3. Specialized mucosa	Dorsal tongue surface

8.1 Fungiform Papillae

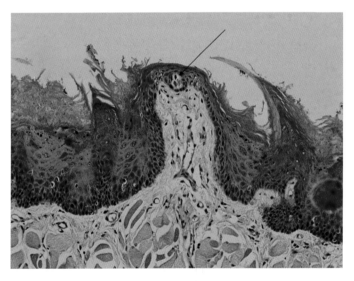

Figure 8.2 H and E stained section showing papillae of the tongue (arrow, taste bud on the superior epithelium of fungiform papilla).

8.1.1 Description

Fungiform papillae are club-shaped/mushroom-shaped and present between the many distributed filiform papillae on the anterior tongue. They usually contain a taste bud on their superior epithelium and their core is made up of connective tissue. Their epithelium could be slightly keratinized or non-keratinized. As compared with the rest of the tongue, their epithelium is thin and their connective tissue is rich in blood supply. Due to this, on clinical examination of the tongue they are seen as red dots or prominences. Their number usually ranges between 200 and 400 near the tip of the tongue but could be different as dorsum of the tongue is affected by many local and systemic factors. Fungiform papillae usually contain taste buds but presence of these without taste buds is also not uncommon.

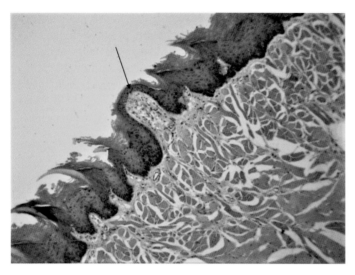

Figure 8.3 H and E stained section showing papillae of the tongue (arrow, superior epithelium of fungiform papilla without taste bud).

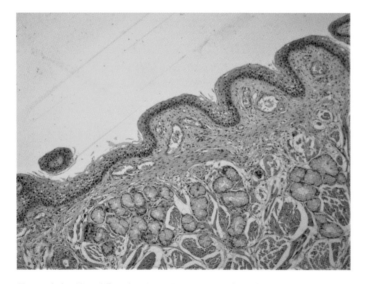

Figure 8.4 H and E stained section showing fungiform papillae of the tongue.

8.1.2 Key Identifying Features

Fungiform papillae appear as fungus or mushroom shaped. A single fungiform papilla is elevated and usually present between many filiform papillae. Taste bud contained within a fungiform papillae appears as a spherical or roughly rounded structure.

8.1.3 Clinical Significance

Fungiform papillae were first defined by Leonard in 1905 [1]. Fungiform papillae are associated with gustatory function and usually contain taste buds in their epithelium [2]. These taste buds could range from 0 to 20 and are responsible to differentiate between diverse taste sensations [3]. In many studies, the count of fungiform papillae has been taken into account to assess an increase or decrease in taste sensitivity [4, 5]. Different techniques and methods like digital photography, contact endoscopy, and use of coloring dye have been proposed in the literature to analyze the count of fungiform papillae [3]. Two important factors that have associated with a decrease in fungiform papillae and consequently taste sensation are nutritional deficiencies and increasing age [3]. Where nutritional deficiencies to some extent can be prevented, inhibiting their decrease with age is still being researched.

8.2 Filiform Papillae

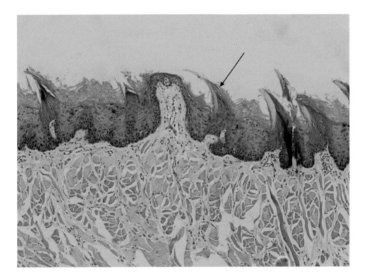

Figure 8.5 H and E stained section showing papillae of the tongue (arrow, filiform papillae).

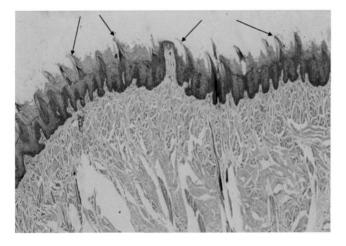

Figure 8.6 H and E stained section showing papillae of the tongue (arrows, filiform papillae).

8.2.1 Description

Filiform papillae are hair-like projections forming a coating on anterior two thirds of the tongue. They start to develop at the 10th week of gestation. They are most numerous on human tongue and are always keratinized. Together with their thick keratinized stratified squamous epithelium and core of connective tissue, filiform papillae form a hard velvety surface of tongue on which the food is compressed and broken down when the tongue is pressed against hard palate. As explained previously, fungiform papilla is dispersed between many filiform papillae. Where fungiform papillae usually contain taste buds, filiform papillae are devoid of any taste buds and are the only non-gustatory papillae of tongue. Cleaning of tongue is very important as bacteria can reside over or under filiform papillae causing bad odor.

8.2.2 Key Identifying Features

The word filiform means "file-like." Filiform papillae appear as filum, elevated threads, or conical hair-like projections on histological sections. They contain a wide base and narrow tip. Their tip could be mostly pointed; however, sometimes a more rounded tip could also be found.

8.2.3 Clinical Significance

Filiform papillae are mechanical papillae (not sensory) which lack nervous elements [6]. Filiform papillae make the tongue rough and give it texture and this feature helps the tongue to grip and process foods [7]. Wong et al. also proposed that they help in moving the food from tongue/oral cavity to esophagus and in distribution of saliva as well [8]. With increasing age and sometimes with nutritional deficiencies, the number of filiform papillae decreases and this gives dorsal surface of the tongue a glossy and smooth appearance [2]. In some patients, keratin covering filiform papillae becomes prominently thick and there is hypertrophy of these papillae, giving the tongue a hairy appearance, a condition called as hairy tongue [2].

8.3 Circumvallate Papilla

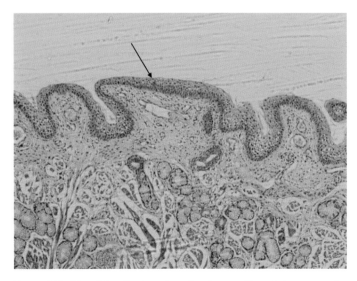

Figure 8.7 H and E stained section showing papillae of the tongue (arrow, circumvallate papilla).

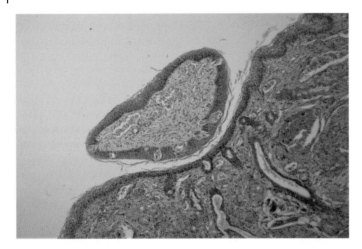

Figure 8.8   H and E stained section showing circumvallate papilla of the tongue.

8.3.1   Description

The word circumvallate means "walled around." These are one of the gustatory papillae of the tongue as they usually contain taste buds. Their number ranges from 8 to 12 and they are located just in front of sulcus terminalis. Their core is made up of connective tissue which is covered on the outside by epithelium (usually keratinized on the top and non-keratinized on lateral walls). These papillae are elevated above the base of the tongue where their smaller portion is attached to it and broader portion is projected above it (but not above the normal level of tongue). They are surrounded by deep groove/trench into which duct of minor salivary gland, i.e. von Ebner gland, opens. Their nerve supply comes from glossopharyngeal nerve even though they are located anterior to foramen caecum and sulcus terminalis (V-shaped groove on dorsal surface of the tongue which parts anterior two thirds of tongue from posterior one third).

8.3.2   Key Identifying Features

Bigger in size and less numerous than filiform and fungiform papillae, they are dome-shaped with raised edges around a depression. Taste buds (if present) are located on the lateral wall of circumvallate papillae.

8.3.3   Clinical Significance

Circumvallate papillae containing taste buds are involved in gustatory sensation [9]. Sometimes minor salivary glands are incorporated inside these papillae and this arrangement helps in the digestion of food [10]. A linear relationship exists between the number of tongue papillae and taste intensity [11]. Aging and certain medical conditions can lead to degeneration of tongue papillae and lead to a partial or complete ageusia [12]. Benign connective tissue disorders and neurological conditions like neurilemmoma or schwannoma also affect the tongue and its papillae and could lead to decreased taste sensation [13].

8.4   Taste Buds

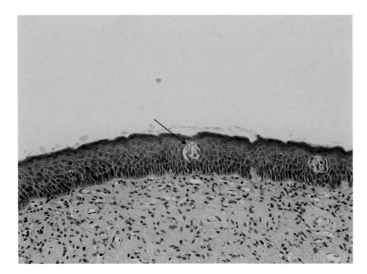

Figure 8.9   H and E stained section (arrow, taste bud).

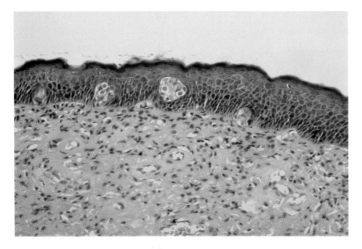

Figure 8.10   H and E stained section showing taste buds.

8.4.1   Description

Taste buds are located on the tongue and help in identification of sweet, salty, sour, bitter, and umami taste sensations. They are located on fungiform, circumvallate, and foliate papillae of tongue. Apart from tongue, they are also located in the mucosa of the soft palate, pharynx, and larynx. Each taste bud contains supporting cells and taste receptor cells (of epithelial origin). The former forms the boundary of the bud whereas the latter is present in the core of the bud. All taste buds are usually composed of 80–100 taste receptor cells which project into a taste pore via a microvilli. Food particles with different tastes are dissolved in the saliva and then carried to taste pores. These dissolved particles do not enter the taste bud; rather they attach to receptors on microvilli in the taste pores. This results in transduction of a gustatory sensation. In this manner, taste cells are similar to neurons as they have the potential to generate action potential. The taste cells of these taste buds have good renewal capability and are replaced after almost every 10 days.

8.4.2 Key Identifying Features

Located on the papillae of the tongue, taste buds are pear-shaped, ovoid, roughly rounded, or spherical structures.

8.4.3 Clinical Significance

The sense of taste is dependent on the presence and accurate functioning of taste buds. These buds are the first stage of taste signaling process and through different cranial nerves (CN), i.e. chorda tympani of facial (VII CN) distributed via lingual nerve (V CN), glossopharyngeal (IX CN), and vagus (X CN), taste signals are transmitted to the brain [14]. The taste buds not only identify nutrients but are also involved in detection of toxins and thus have a protective role as well [15]. The normal aging process and certain disorders (Sjögren's syndrome, oral cancer, Parkinson's disease, and Alzheimer's disease) can disturb the turnover rate of taste cells and hence can affect the quality of life by causing malnutrition and weight loss [15–18]. Certain habits like smoking can also affect somatosensory function in tongue [19].

8.5 Keratinized Oral Epithelium

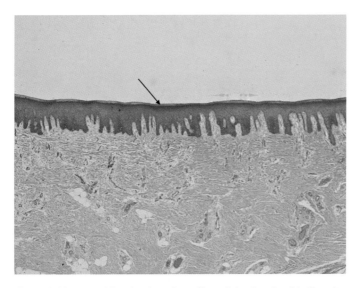

Figure 8.11 H and E stained section of keratinized oral epithelium (arrow, keratin layer).

8.5.1 Description

Masticatory mucosa present on the hard palate, attached gingiva, and dorsal surface of the tongue is rigid and tough and is composed of keratinized stratified squamous epithelium. Keratinization also called as cornification is a process that makes the outer surface hard and resilient to abrasion. The size of keratinization depends on the magnitude of stress induced on the surface. Keratinized oral epithelium consists of four distinct layer of cells, i.e. basal layer (stratum basale), prickle layer (stratum spinosum), granular layer (stratum granulosum), and keratinized surface layer (stratum corneum). The maturing pattern of these cells is called ortho-keratinization. The shape of the cells in these layers is different with basal layer cells being cuboidal or columnar, prickle layer cells being spherical, granular layer consisting of cells being flattened with keratohyalin granules, and surface keratin layer cells (keratinocytes) being squamous or squames-like without any nuclei. The oral epithelium is connected with the underlying connective tissue or lamina propria with an irregular interface. This interface is based on finger-like projections where projections of epithelium into connective tissue are called rete pegs whereas the projections of connective tissue into epithelium are called connective tissue papillae.

8.5.2 Key Identifying Features

A distinctive keratin layer without any nuclei on the surface of epithelium. Appears bright pink on hematoxylin and eosin staining. The thickness of keratin layer is variable, being different in different individuals.

8.5.3 Clinical Significance

Keratin is an aggregation of proteins which are joined together by disulphide bonds providing the layer with its characteristic mechanical and chemical strength [20]. Keratins can impact mitotic activity of epithelial cells [21]. The only other biological material which has comparable toughness to keratin is chitin [22]. The main function of keratinized epithelial layer is to protect underlying mucosa and deeper tissues from the environment [23]. Abnormalities related to keratinization are also not very uncommon and are classified generally as hyperkeratinization, hypokeratinization, or abnormal keratinization [21].

8.6 Parakeratinized Oral Epithelium

8.6.1 Description

Parakeratinized oral epithelium is similar to keratinized epithelium in many aspects as it also contains four distinct layer of cells, i.e. basal layer (stratum basale), prickle layer (stratum spinosum), granular layer (stratum granulosum), and keratinized surface layer (stratum corneum). The shape of cells in these layers of parakeratinized epithelium is almost similar to keratinized

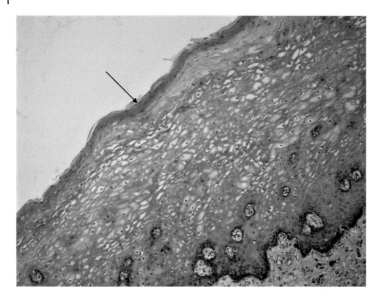

Figure 8.12 H and E stained section of parakeratinized oral epithelium (arrow, keratin layer with pykontic nuclei).

epithelium as well. However, masticatory mucosa sometimes shows a variation in the degree of keratinization. One type of variation in which keratin layer is present but with pyknotic nuclei inside squames is called parakeratinization. The parakeratinized epithelium can contain keratohyalin granules in its granular layer but they may be few, dispersed, and less pronounced than in orthokeratinized epithelium. This is why the parakeratinized epithelium has ill-defined stratum granulosum. Parakeratinized epithelium is found mostly in parts of gingiva where around 75% of it is parakeratinized.

8.6.2 Key Identifying Features

Parakeratinized epithelium generally refers to partial or incomplete keratinization of stratum corneum. It is described by a distinctive keratin layer with retained nuclei at the uppermost surface. Keratin layer appears bright pink on H and E staining with condensed and flattened nuclei.

8.6.3 Clinical Significance

Parakeratinization of oral mucosa is considered a normal process and is unlike epidermis where parakeratinization could be a sign of a disease [24]. Just similar to keratinized epithelium, its function is also to act as a tough protective barrier for deeper tissues and prevent any chemical or mechanical injury [25]. The presence of rete pegs and connective tissue papillae ensures firm attachment of epithelium with lamina propria, hence superimposing its function to act as a strong barrier against chemical or mechanical injuries [26].

8.7 Non-Keratinized Oral Epithelium

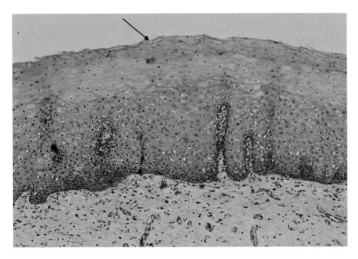

Figure 8.13   H and E stained section of keratinized oral epithelium (arrow, superior surface without keratin layer).

8.7.1 Description

Non-keratinized stratified squamous epithelium is present as a lining mucosa in many parts of the oral cavity which includes lips, ventral surface of tongue, buccal mucosa, and soft palate. It lacks a keratin layer also termed as cornified surface layer but the epithelium thickness is more than the keratinized epithelium. In terms of structural hierarchy, basal and prickle layers are similar to keratinized epithelium despite the fact that the cells of non-keratinized epithelium are marginally greater in dimensions. For this reason, many researchers avoid the term "prickle cell layer" for non-keratinized epithelium and describe it as having basal layer (stratum basale), intermedium layer (stratum intermedium), and superficial layer (stratum superficiale). It should be noted here that non-keratinized epithelium does not contain any granular layer (stratum granulosum) with keratohyalin granules. The cells of the top layer contain nuclei but they do not stain strongly with eosin as the keratin layer does in keratinized and parakeratinized oral epithelium.

8.7.2 Key Identifying Features

An epithelial layer containing flattened nuclei at the superior surface but lacks a keratin layer. Rete pegs and connective tissue papillae are although present, but they show less well-defined assembly or are usually shorter if compared with keratinized epithelium.

8.7.3 Clinical Significance

Non-keratinized epithelium is present in areas where there are less forces directed or less mastica-tory pressures [21]. This is the most accepted reason for the absence of keratin layer at the superior surface of non-keratinized epithelium [1]. Depending on the stimuli induced, non-keratinized epithelium can be converted into keratinized epithelium and the term used for such a transition is keratosis [27].

8.8 Non-Specific Ulcer

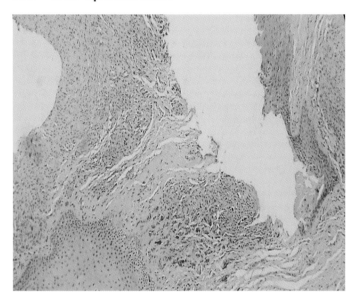

Figure 8.14 H and E stained section of the tissue showing deep ulcer with dense chronic inflammation extending into deep underlying connective tissue.

8.8.1 Description

Ulcerations are marked by epithelial lesions or the connective tissue underlying them or both. Because of the heterogeneity of causative factors and symptoms, it can be very difficult to diagnose oral ulcerative lesions. The traumatic mucosal ulcer is a common self-limited oral condition that clinically presents as solitary ulceration with sharp, punched-out pale indurated borders that affect the tongue, buccal mucosa, or lip. It usually affects older adults but may occur at any age, including children, and may or may not be painful. These ulcers are often self-healing, but many may persist for weeks or longer. The cause is usually unknown but trauma is usually associated with them.

8.8.2 Key Identifying Features

Microscopically there is usually a deep ulcer with associated dense acute and chronic inflammation extending into deep underlying tissue, sometimes involving voluntary muscle. The infiltrate includes numerous lymphocytes and eosinophils, together with some normal histiocytes.

8.8.3 Clinical Considerations

The ulcers often spontaneously heal after the biopsy; however, their recurrence is common, particularly if there is persistent trauma [28]. Where there is associated atypical epithelial hyperplasia, clinical follow-up is important to exclude the possibility of a developing malignancy [29].

8.9 Oral Lichen Planus

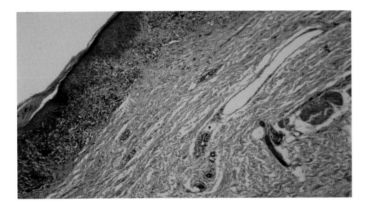

Figure 8.15 H and E stained section showing hyperkeratosis, subepithelial band of lymphocytic infiltration, sawtooth-shaped rete ridges, and deeper connective tissue free of inflammation.

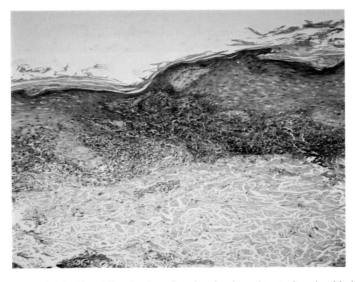

Figure 8.16 H and E stained section showing hyperkeratosis, subepithelial band of lymphocytic infiltration, sawtooth-shaped rete ridges, and deeper connective tissue free of inflammation.

8.9.1 Description

Lichen planus is a chronic inflammatory autoimmune condition that affects both the skin and the mucus membranes. The lichen planus is the mucosal counterpart of dermatological lichen planus which affects 1–2% of the population. It typically affects people over the age of 45, with an average incidence between 50 and 60 years of age, but it may also affect children and adolescents. It is more prevalent among women than men (1.4 : 1). Clinically, it can be divided as having the different types like reticular, papular, plaque-like, erosive, atrophic, or bullous. Intraoral involvement is often seen in the buccal mucosa, tongue, and gingiva even though it is rare for other areas. Oral mucosal lesions are present either alone or with concurrent skin lesions. It is an autoimmune-mediated T-cell disease in which the auto-cytotoxic CD8 + T cells stimulate apoptosis of oral epithelium's basal cells and the reticular form is the most prevalent type of oral planus lichen. This shows white keratotic interlacing lines with an erythematous margin traditionally known as Wickham's striae. Usually, these striae are present bilaterally on the buccal mucosa. The second most common type of oral lichen planus is the erosive type. This provides a combination of erythematous and ulcerated areas surrounded by fine keratotic strewing striae. The atrophic and bullous types are two additional presentations, which are deemed variants of the erosive lichen planus. Atrophic lichen planus appears as diffused, erythematous patches surrounded by tiny white striae. This type of lichen planus can cause severe pain and burning discomfort. In the bullous type of lichen planus, intraoral bullae are found on the buccal mucosa and the tongue's lateral borders; the bullae breach open shortly after they appear, resulting in the classic appearance of erosive lichen planus.

8.9.2 Key Identifying Features

The definitive diagnosis of oral lichen planus is determined by histopathological analysis. The classic histopathologic features include hyperkeratosis, basal cell degeneration, thick subepithelial band of lymphocytic infiltration, sawtooth-shaped rete ridges, and deeper connective tissue which is free of inflammation.

8.9.3 Clinical Considerations

Oral lichen planus is one of the most prevalent mucosal diseases that affect the oral cavity [30]. Thus, dentists regularly encounter patients with this condition in daily clinical practice. Since patients usually experience significant discomfort with the atrophic and erosive types of oral lichen planus, knowledge of the available treatment protocols is critical [31]. The similarity between oral lichen planus and many other vesiculobullous-ulcerative disorders, some of which may result in severe morbidity, makes accurate diagnosis vital [32]. Several findings indicate an elevated risk of squamous cell carcinoma in patients suffering from oral lichen planus lesions [33, 34]. Apparently, there is no treatment for oral lichen planus and the treatment and care are mainly intended to reduce symptomatic disease duration and severity [35]. The most widely known treatment for oral lichen planus lesions includes topical or systemic corticosteroids, which modulates the immune response of the patient [31]. The prognosis of oral lichen planus is not clear as it can be resolved within a few months, or it can linger for decades, with or without medication [36]. Often there are periods of remission and relapse [36].

8.10 Pemphigoid

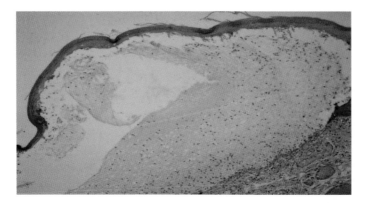

Figure 8.17 H and E stained section of the tissue showing subepithelial vesicle formation and a split (the epithelium is segregated from the connective tissue at basement membrane zone).

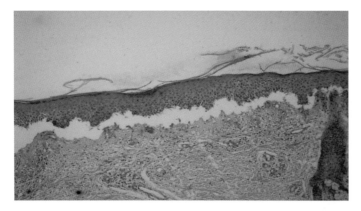

Figure 8.18 H and E stained section of the tissue showing subepithelial vesicle formation and a split (the epithelium is segregated from the connective tissue at basement membrane zone).

8.10.1 Description

Pemphigoid is an indiscriminate group of chronic autoimmune subepithelial vesiculobullous conditions that primarily affects the mucosa and often the skin as well. It is marked by the presence of autoantibodies against distinct structural components of the dermal–epidermal junction. Pemphigoid occurs mostly in elderly people (mid 60s) and women are more affected than men. The etiology of this condition is unclear. A genetic association has been identified which suggests the role for antigen recognition of T-lymphocytes in the epithelial basement membrane zone and the IgG and/or IgA autoantibodies against different hemidesmosomic components are responsible for the development of subepithelial blisters. The presence of oral lesions is the main clinical sign and they can occur all over the oral mucosa. Taut, serous, or hemorrhagic blisters quickly get ruptured by mechanical forces and contribute to irregular erosions or yellowish slough ulcers surrounded by the erythematous halo.

8.10.2 Key Identifying Features

The characteristic histopathologic features include a subepithelial vesicle formation and a split (the epithelium is segregated from the connective tissue at the basement membrane zone). The epithelium is intact without acantholysis and connective tissue can show some degree of inflammatory cell infiltration.

8.10.3 Clinical Considerations

Pemphigoid is a chronic disorder characterized by exacerbations and remissions over months to years. Symptoms may include pain, dysphagia, soreness, foetor, mucosal bleeding, and/or mucosal peeling [37]. The treatment of choice is systemic corticosteroids and immunosuppressants [37]. However, in some patients the disease is self-limiting, resulting in disease remissions within a few years [38]. Pemphigoid is a chronic progressive disease that could change into a life-threatening condition (such as those with airway involvement) [38]. The involvement of multiple erosions and immunosuppressive drugs used to manage the disease may cause secondary infections and such infections can either be localized to mucosa alone or could result in systemic changes [38].

8.11 Lipoma

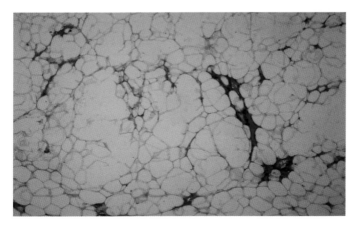

Figure 8.19 H and E stained section showing round/ovoid mature fat cells appearing empty without cytoplasm and crescent-shaped pyknotic nuclei pushed to the periphery.

8.11.1 Description

Lipomas are the most common benign soft tissue tumors that are composed chiefly of adipose tissue. Approximately 20% of them occur in the area of head and neck and oral lipomas comprise about 1–4% of all the cases. In the oral cavity, it is most commonly located in the cheeks, floor of the mouth, and the tongue. Lipoma has also been called as a "yellow epulis" because when it is located in the superficial plane, there is a yellow surface discoloration. The tumor has a less dense and more uniform appearance than surrounding fibrovascular tissues when it is transilluminated.

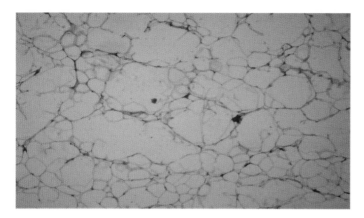

Figure 8.20 H and E stained section showing round/ovoid mature fat cells appearing empty without cytoplasm and crescent-shaped pyknotic nuclei pushed to the periphery.

8.11.2 Key Identifying Features

The histopathologic features comprise of round to ovoid mature fat cells. These cells appear empty without cytoplasm and the nucleus is pushed to the periphery. The crescent-shaped pyknotic nucleus is a pathognomic of lipoma. The lesion is well-circumscribed and may have a connective tissue capsule. Connective tissue septa are often seen dividing the lesion into many lobules.

8.11.3 Clinical Considerations

Lipomas are asymptomatic, slow-growing, and could be present for several years [39]. Magnetic resonance imaging (MRI) scans are very useful in diagnosis whereas computed tomography (CT) and ultrasound scans are less reliable [39]. Irrespective of their location, the treatment is simple surgical excision, including a cuff of surrounding tissue to prevent local recurrences [40]. Advantages of suction-abetted lipectomy have been recognized and reported for medium-sized (4–10 cm) or large lipomas (>10 cm) [39]. To retain as much normal tissue as possible, an infiltrating lipoma must be "de-bulked" where a part of the infiltrating fat is intentionally left untouched [41]. In the oral and maxillofacial region, malignant changes or recurrences are rare [42].

8.12 Oral Epithelial Dysplasia

8.12.1 Description

Oral cancer is one of the diseases with highest mortality rate. The majority of cases of oral cancer are linked to certain behaviors such as tobacco and areca nut consumption. It is followed by clinical asymptomatic lesions generally known as potentially malignant disorders (PMDs). It is a clinical diagnosis for which hyperkeratosis, hyperplasia, oral epithelial dysplasia, or oral squamous cell carcinoma (OSCC) constitute the features of histopathological diagnosis. Oral epithelial dysplasia is the earliest form of these oral PMDs. The word "dysplasia" denotes abnormal growth. This term is applied to early cellular changes associated with an increased risk of malignant potential, often called "atypia." Epithelial dysplasia is categorized as mild, moderate, severe, and carcinoma *in-situ*. Differentiation is made between mild, moderate, and severe based on a histopathological

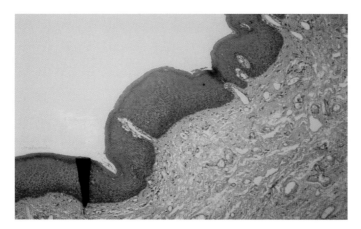

Figure 8.21 H and E stained section of the tissue showing mild epithelial dysplasia with different architectural and cellular dysplastic changes.

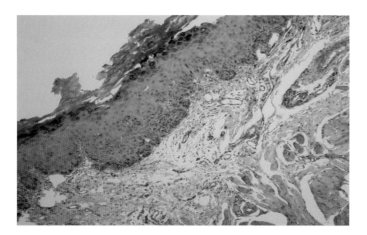

Figure 8.22 H and E stained section of the tissue showing moderate epithelial dysplasia with different architectural and cellular dysplastic changes.

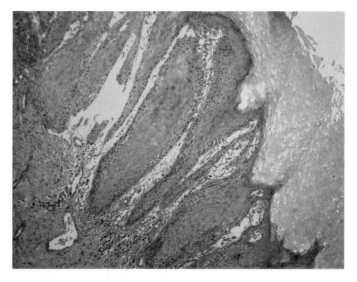

Figure 8.23 H and E stained section of the tissue showing severe epithelial dysplasia with different architectural and cellular dysplastic changes.

investigation through to the presence and severity of cellular atypia and the architectural altera-tions. When the tumor starts to invade the surrounding tissue, the epithelial dysplasia converts to micro-invasive SCC. The dysplastic changes/alterations are categorized into cellular alterations followed by architectural alterations. In the former, there is anisonucleosis, anisocytosis, nuclear pleomorphism, cellular pleomorphism, increased nuclear-cytoplasmic ratio, increased number and size of nucleoli, dyskeratosis, and atypical mitotic figures. In the latter, there is irregular epi-thelial stratification, loss of polarity of basal cells, drop-shaped rete ridges, keratin pearls within rete pegs, abnormally superficial mitosis, and increased number of mitotic figures.

8.12.2 Key Identifying Features

The execution of these alterations should be done bearing in mind the epithelium is divided into "thirds." Accordingly, the lesions should therefore be graded into: *Mild dysplasia*, architectural changes along with cellular atypia is noted only in the lower third part of the epithelium; *Moderate dysplasia*, architectural changes extending into the middle third of the epithelium constitutes moder-ate dysplasia, but the degree of cellular atypia is required for upgrading it to "severe dysplasia"; *Severe dysplasia*, architectural changes affecting greater than two-thirds of the epithelium, along with cel-lular atypical changes. Carcinoma *in situ* which demonstrates that there is a malignant transforma-tion, but the invasion has not taken place and it could be the next stage after severe dysplasia.

8.12.3 Clinical Considerations

About 5–18% of all epithelial dysplasias become malignant [43]. The histopathological evaluation for the existence of epithelial dysplasia is known as the "touchstone" for predicting malignant trans-formation of PMDs [44]. A vital indicator of the malignancy potential of these conditions is the histopathological existence of epithelial dysplasia [43]. The more severe the degree of dysplasia, greater the possibility of malignant transformation, is expected [45]. The treatment of choice for oral cavity epithelial dysplasia is the scalpel or a CO_2 laser-assisted surgical excision [46]. The laser offers a relatively bloodless operating environment and shows a decreased risk of recurrence [46]. It should be noted that delayed diagnosis impedes effective treatment and beneficial outcomes.

8.13 Oral Melanoma

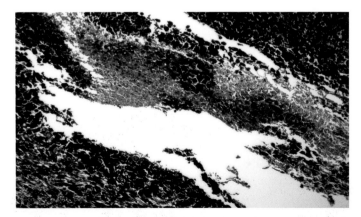

Figure 8.24 H and E stained section showing diffused proliferation of neoplastic melanocytes with atrophic stratified squamous epithelium and chronic inflammatory cells.

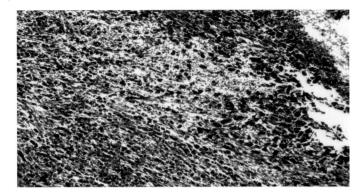

Figure 8.25 H and E stained section showing diffused proliferation of neoplastic melanocytes with atrophic stratified squamous epithelium and chronic inflammatory cells.

8.13.1 Description

Melanoma is a malignant tumor which is composed of melanocytes. In melanoma, the cells are produced from neural crest that makes up the melanin pigment in the epithelium's basal and supra-basilar layers. While most melanomas occur in the skin, they can emerge from mucosal surfaces as well. Oral malignant melanomas are somewhat rare tumors (representing about 2% of all melanomas). The etiology of melanoma is not clear but some of the possible risk factors are cigarette smoking, denture sensitivity, and alcohol intake, but their association is still unsubstantiated. The development of malignant melanomas typically occurs between the ages of 40 and 70 years, with a median age of 55 years. Melanoma is three times more common among males than females and malignant melanomas are most common in the palate and maxilla. Oral melanoma is initially asymptomatic, and develops unnoticed by patients, leading to diagnostic delays. Recognition of the lesion usually occurs when the overlying epithelium is deteriorated or when there is an occurrence of hemorrhage. Melanomas can vary with or without ulcerations from coral pink over brown and blue to black lesions. They may be flat or raised along an erythematous border around the lesion.

8.13.2 Key Identifying Features

Histopathological findings of oral melanoma indicate the presence of large, round-to-oval epithelioid melanocytes with atrophic stratified squamous epithelium. The stroma of the connective tissue reflects the diffuse proliferation of neoplastic, round-to-oval melanocytes, with chronic inflammatory cells.

8.13.3 Clinical Considerations

Oral melanomas are characterized by pronounced aggressive and invasive behavior, which spreads to locations such as lungs, liver, brain, and bones through both local and distant metastasis [47]. A key prognostic factor for oral melanomas appears to be the lymphatic metastasis at the time of diagnosis [48]. Surgery, along with chemotherapy, radiotherapy, and immunotherapy, remains the standard treatment [48]. Recent surgical excision accompanied by immuno-chemotherapy has been shown to have decreased or stopped the lesion completely from recurring [49]. Despite a five-year survival rate of 0–55% of cases, oral melanoma has a poor prognosis. With any oral mucosal melanomas, the median survival is significantly more than two years after diagnosis [50]. These tumors are clinically very quiet and asymptomatic and seem to be deceptive and thus the significance of early detection and treatment that can be lifesaving cannot be overemphasized.

References

1 Leonard, T.M.R. (1905). Ankylostomiasis or uncinariasis. *JAMA* 45: 588–594.

2 Nanci, A. and Ten, C.A.R. (2003). *Ten Cate's Oral Histology: Development, Structure, and Function.* St. Louis, MO: Mosby.

3 Khan, A., Ali, S., Jameela, R.V. et al. (2019). Impact of fungiform papillae count on taste perception and different methods of taste assessment and their clinical applications: a comprehensive review. *Sultan Qaboos University Med J* 19 (3): e184–e191.

4 Pavlidis, P., Gouveris, H., and Kekes, G. (2017). Electrogustometry thresholds, tongue tip vascularization, density, and form of the fungiform papillae following smoking cessation. *Chem Senses* 42: 419–423.

5 Nasri-Heir, C., Gomes, J., Heir, G.M. et al. (2011). The role of sensory input of the chorda tympani nerve and the number of fungiform papillae in burning mouth syndrome. *Oral Surg Oral Med Oral Pathol Oral Radiol Endod* 112: 65–72.

6 Sato, O., Maeda, T., Kobayashi, S. et al. (1988). Filiform papillae as a sensory apparatus in the tongue: an immunohistochemical study of nervous elements by use of neurofilament protein (NFP) and S-100 protein antibodies. *Cell Tissue Res* 252 (2): 231–238.

7 Kawasaki, M., Kawasaki, K., Oommen, S. et al. (2016). Regional regulation of Filiform tongue papillae development by Ikkα/Irf6. *Dev Dyn* 245 (9): 937–946.

8 Wong, P., Colucci-Guyon, E., Takahashi, K. et al. (2000). Introducing a null mutation in the mouse K6alpha and K6beta genes reveals their essential structural role in the oral mucosa. *J Cell Biol* 150: 921–928.

9 Sbarbati, A., Crescimanno, C., and Osculati, F. (1999). The anatomy and functional role of the circumvallate papilla/von Ebner gland complex. *Med Hypotheses* 53 (1): 40–44.

10 Matsuo, R. (2000). Role of saliva in the maintenance of taste sensitivity. *Crit Rev Oral Biol Med* 11 (2): 216–229.

11 Walliczek-Dworschak, U., Schöps, F., Feron, G. et al. (2017). Differences in the density of fungiform papillae and composition of saliva in patients with taste disorders compared to healthy controls. *Chem Senses* 42 (8): 699–708.

12 Heckmann, J.G., Heckmann, S.M., Lang, C.J., and Hummel, T. (2003). Neurological aspects of taste disorders. *Arch Neurol* 60 (5): 667–671.

13 Brito, J.A.R., Souza, F.T.A., Lacerda, J.C.T. et al. (2012). Asymptomatic nodule in the tongue. *Oral Surg Oral Med Oral Pathol Oral Radiol* 114: 281–283.

14 Breslin, P.A. (2013). An evolutionary perspective on food and human taste. *Curr Biol* 23 (9): R409–R418.

15 Feng, P., Huang, L., and Wang, H. (2014). Taste bud homeostasis in health, disease, and aging. *Chem Senses* 39 (1): 3–16.

16 Heft, M.W. and Robinson, M.E. (2010). Age differences in orofacial sensory thresholds. *J Dent Res* 89: 1102–1105.

17 Carson, J.A. and Gormican, A. (1977). Taste acuity and food attitudes of selected patients with cancer. *J Am Diet Assoc* 70: 361–365.

18 Kashihara, K., Hanaoka, A., and Imamura, T. (2011). Frequency and characteristics of taste impairment in patients with Parkinson's disease: results of a clinical interview. *Intern Med* 50: 2311–2315.

19 Yekta, S.S., Lückhoff, A., Ristić, D. et al. (2012). Impaired somatosensation in tongue mucosa of smokers. *Clin Oral Investig* 16 (1): 39–44.

20 McKittrick, J., Chen, P.-Y., Bodde, G. et al. (2012). The structure, functions, and mechanical properties of keratin. *JOM* 64 (4): 449–468.

21 Deo, P.N. and Deshmukh, R. (2018). Pathophysiology of keratinization. *J Oral Maxillofac Pathol* 22: 86–91.

22 Vincent, J.F. and Wegst, U.G. (2004). Design and mechanical properties of insect cuticle. *Arthropod Struct Dev* 33 (3): 187–199.

23 Bragulla, H.H. and Homberger, D.G. (2009). Structure and functions of keratin proteins in simple, stratified, keratinized and cornified epithelia. *J Anat* 214 (4): 516–559.

24 Bloor, B.K., Tidman, N., Leigh, I.M. et al. (2003). Expression of keratin K2e in cutaneous and oral lesions: association with keratinocyte activation, proliferation, and keratinization. *Am J Pathol* 162 (3): 963–975.

25 Groeger, S. and Meyle, J. (2019). Oral mucosal epithelial cells. *Front Immunol* 10: 208.

26 Groeger, S.E. and Meyle, J. (2015). Epithelial barrier and oral bacterial infection. *Periodontol 2000* 69 (1): 46–67.

27 Bhaskar, S.N. and Orban, B.J. (1991). *Orban's Oral Histology and Embryology*. St. Louis: Mosby Year Book.

28 Dhanrajani, P. and Cropley, P.W. (2015). Oral eosinophilic or traumatic ulcer: a case report and brief review. *Natl J Maxillofac Surg* 6 (2): 237–240. https://doi.org/10.4103/0975-5950.183854.

29 Gagari, E., Stathopoulos, P., Katsambas, A., and Avgerinou, G. (2011). Traumatic ulcerative granuloma with stromal eosinophilia: a lesion with alarming histopathologic presentation and benign clinical course. *Am J Dermatopathol* 33: 192–194.

30 Pynn, B.R., Burgess, K.L., Wade, P.S., and McComb, R.J. (1995). A retrospective survey of 2021 patients referred to the Toronto Hospital Mouth Clinic. *Ont Dent* 72 (1): 21–24.

31 Lavanya, N., Jayanthi, P., Rao, U.K., and Ranganathan, K. (2011). Oral lichen planus: an update on pathogenesis and treatment. *J Oral Maxillofac Pathol* 15 (2): 127–132.

32 Gupta, S. and Jawanda, M.K. (2015). Oral lichen planus: an update on etiology, pathogenesis, clinical presentation, diagnosis and management. *Indian J Dermatol* 60 (3): 222–229.

33 Silverman, S. Jr. and Bahl, S. (1997). Oral lichen planus update: clinical characteristics, treatment responses, and malignant transformation. *Am J Dent* 10 (6): 259–263. 18.

34 Barnard, N.A., Scully, C., Eveson, J.W. et al. (1993). Oral cancer development in patients with oral lichen planus. *J Oral Pathol Med* 22 (9): 421–424.

35 Mostafa, D., Moussa, E., and Alnouaem, M. (2017). Evaluation of photodynamic therapy in treatment of oral erosive lichen planus in comparison with topically applied corticosteroids. *Photodiagnosis Photodyn Ther* 19: 56–66.

36 Kaplan, I., Ventura-Sharabi, Y., Gal, G. et al. (2012). The dynamics of oral lichen planus: a retrospective clinicopathological study. *Head Neck Pathol* 6 (2): 178–183.

37 Hammers, C.M. and Stanley, J.R. (2016). Mechanisms of disease: pemphigus and bullous pemphigoid. *Annu Rev Pathol* 11: 175–197.

38 Han, A. (2009). A practical approach to treating autoimmune bullous disorders with systemic medications. *J Clin Aesthet Dermatol* 2 (5): 19–28.

39 Mohammed, F., Fairozekhan, T.A., Mohamed, S. et al. (2013). Yellow lesions of the oral cavity: diagnostic appraisal and management strategies. *Brunei Int Med J* 9 (5): 290–301.

40 Amber, K.T., Ovadia, S., and Camacho, I. (2014). Injection therapy for the management of superficial subcutaneous lipomas. *J Clin Aesthet Dermatol* 7 (6): 46–48.

41 Epivatianos, A., Markopoulos, A.K., and Papanayotou, P. (2000). Benign tumors of adipose tissue of the oral cavity: a clinicopathologic study of 13 cases. *J Oral Maxillofac Surg* 58: 1113–1117.

42 Bandéca, M.C., de Pádua, J.M., Nadalin, M.R. et al. (2007). Oral soft tissue lipomas: a case series. *JCDA* 73: 5.

43 Axell, T., Pindborg, J.J., Smith, C.J., and van der Waal, I. (1996). Oral white lesions with special reference to precancerous and tobacco-related lesions: conclusions of an international symposium held in Uppsala, Sweden, 1994. *J Oral Pathol Med* 25: 49–54.

44 UEG Week (2015). Oral presentations. *United European Gastroenterol J* 3 (5 Suppl): 1–145.

45 Ranganathan, K. and Kavitha, L. (2019). Oral epithelial dysplasia: classifications and clinical relevance in risk assessment of oral potentially malignant disorders. *J Oral Maxillofac Pathol* 23 (1): 19–27.

46 Monteiro, L., Delgado, M.L., Garcês, F. et al. (2019). A histological evaluation of the surgical margins from human oral fibrous-epithelial lesions excised with CO2 laser, diode laser, Er:YAG laser, Nd:YAG laser, electrosurgical scalpel and cold scalpel. *Med Oral Patol Oral Cir Bucal* 24 (2): e271–e280.

47 Martinez, E.A., Alonso, F.C., and Siles, M.S. (2005). Melanoma of the oral mucosa with cerebral metastasis: a clinical case. *Oral Oncol Extra* 41: 30–33.

48 Zbytek, B., Carlson, J.A., Granese, J. et al. (2008). Current concepts of metastasis in melanoma. *Expert Rev Dermatol* 3 (5): 569–585.

49 Algazi, A.P., Soon, C.W., and Daud, A.I. (2010). Treatment of cutaneous melanoma: current approaches and future prospects. *Cancer Manag Res* 2: 197–211.

50 Chidzonga, M.M., Mahomva, L., Marimo, C., and Makunike-Mutasa, R. (2007). Primary malignant melanoma of the oral mucosa. *J Oral Maxillofac Surg* 65: 1117–1120.

9

Salivary Glands

Fizza Saher[1], Zohaib Khurshid[2], Muhammad Sohail Zafar[3,4], Faraz Mohammed[5], and Syed Ali Khurram[6]

[1] Department of Oral Biology, College of Dentistry, Ziauddin University, Karachi, Pakistan
[2] Department of Prosthodontics and Dental Implantology, College of Dentistry, King Faisal University, Al Ahsa, Saudi Arabia
[3] Department of Restorative Dentistry, College of Dentistry, Taibah University, Al Madinah, Al Munawwarah, Saudi Arabia
[4] Department of Dental Materials, Islamic International Dental College, Riphah International University, Islamabad, Pakistan
[5] Department of Biomedical Dental Sciences, College of Dentistry, Imam Abdulrahman Bin Faisal University, Dammam, Saudi Arabia
[6] Unit of Oral and Maxillofacial Pathology, School of Clinical Dentistry, University of Sheffield, Sheffield, United Kingdom

The oral cavity has a dynamic moist environment from the embryonic stage till the end of life. This unique environment encounters many microbial and pathogen attacks. To defend it, specialized oral epithelium lining and salivary glands play a crucial role [1]. The parotid, submandibular, and sublingual glands are the highly specialized functional major salivary glands and they perform an essential role in saliva production [2]. These glands are surrounded by an uneven tight connective tissue sheath which enters into the glands to form septa, and these septa divide the glands into compartments. These compartments might be acinus or tubules or both according to the nature of the gland. Other minor glands of the oral cavity are buccal, labial, glossopalatine, palatine, and lingual glands. The further description of the glands is illustrated in Figure 9.1.

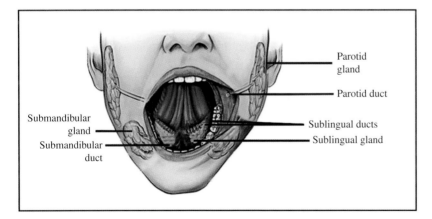

Figure 9.1 Illustration representing the major salivary glands of the oral cavity with their duct openings. *Source:* From ref. [3]. © 2018 Reprinted with permission of Elsevier.

An Illustrated Guide to Oral Histology, First Edition. Edited by Imran Farooq, Saqib Ali, and Paul Anderson.
© 2021 John Wiley & Sons Ltd. Published 2021 by John Wiley & Sons Ltd.
Companion website: www.wiley.com/go/farooq/oral_histology

Human saliva acts as a lubricant with a potent line of defense because of its antibacterial, anti-fungal, and antioxidant properties [4–6]. Whole mouth saliva (WMS) is a blend of salivary gland secretions (major/minor), gingival crevicular fluid (GCF), desquamated oral epithelial cells, and microorganisms [7, 8]. The main ingredients of the secreted saliva include a range of electrolytes, including potassium, bicarbonates, and magnesium [4]. Also, proteins and peptides found in saliva are defensins, cathelicidins, histatins, adrenomedullin, statherin, and neuropeptides [1, 9–11]. Saliva is an exocrine secretion which exchanges through both intracellular and extracellular passageways in the oral cavity. Strikingly, small or nano biomolecules may enter saliva from serum or blood through the capillary barriers, interstitial spaces, and the membranes of the acinar/ductal cells. This complex routes secretion of the saliva, making it an active diagnostic medium for disease detection such as oral cancer, dental caries, periodontal diseases, oral lichen planus, oral squamous cell carcinoma (OSCC), breast cancer, lung cancer, cardiovascular disease, and arthritis [3, 12–14]. Recently, salivary secretion has been approved for the detection of novel coronavirus disease 2019 (COVID-19) or severe acute respiratory syndrome coronavirus 2 (SARS-CoV-2) [15]. In the past, salivary biomarkers were used for the detection of the viruses such as the Zika virus, human papillomavirus (HPV), human immunodeficiency virus (HIV), and hepatitis C virus [16, 17].

The human salivary glands have a complex anatomy. Their common histological features along with some common salivary gland pathologies are discussed in detail in the following sections.

9.1 Serous Salivary Gland

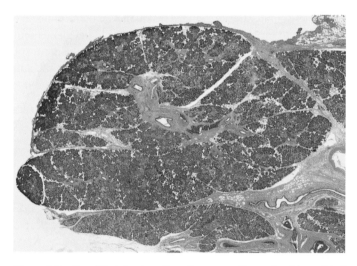

Figure 9.2 H and E stained section of serous salivary gland (parotid gland).

9.1.1 Description

Serous gland cells present with prominent round-shaped nuclei that are located in the basal third of the cell, which is basophilic (because of the abundance of the rough endoplasmic reticulum). In terms of ducts, the serous glands have long intercalated ducts and short striated ducts. The intercalated ducts are lined by cuboidal-shaped epithelial cells that have lumina higher than the acini.

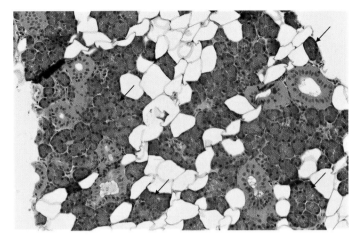

Figure 9.3 H and E stained section of serous salivary gland (arrows, serous acini).

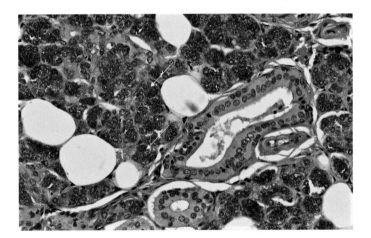

Figure 9.4 H and E stained section of serous salivary gland (arrows, serous acini).

The striated ducts are smaller mucinous glands compared to serous salivary glands. The striation is formed due to the infolding of the basal plasma membrane. The parotid gland is serous and its duct is called Stenson's duct which opens in the oral cavity adjacent to the maxillary second molar tooth. This duct channels the serous secretion from the gland into the oral cavity. Another example of serous gland are the Von Ebner glands which are found in the trough surrounding cicumvallate papillae on the posterolateral surface of the tongue. These are gustatory glands with a role in taste sensation and are the only serious minor glands in the oral cavity.

9.1.2 Key Identifying Features

On histological sections, the cells of the serous salivary gland appear darker. The reason behind their darker histological appearance when stained is their watery secretion that contains a lot of proteins. These cells have a characteristic granular appearance with a wedge-shaped outline, the basal surface being broader, and surround the central lumen. The cell membrane shows numerous microvilli and infoldings. The basal part of each serous cell is delineated from the adjacent connective tissue by a basal lamina.

9.1.3 Clinical Significance and Considerations

The serous glands are responsible for producing smooth secretion of the protein [2]. Their ducts are narrow than the mucous glands [18]. The parotid gland is a large gland that produces most of the saliva, and its flow is disturbed by the use of certain drugs, or under certain conditions like stress, bacterial infection, and the presence of stones in the secretory ducts. The parotitis is an inflammatory condition of the parotid glands that may affect a person unilaterally or bilaterally [19]. The parotitis could be caused by a virus such as paramyxovirus (mumps), coxsackievirus, influenza A, parainfluenza viruses, and Epstein–Barr virus, and due to an infection by certain bacterial species (*Staphylococcus aureus*, *Streptococcus* species, and gram-negative bacteria) [20]. The infections related to bilateral gland swelling include viral mumps, HIV, acute suppurative parotitis, tuberculosis, and bilateral parotid abscess. The leading etiology of parotitis is mumps. *Streptococcus* species, *S. aureus*, and, infrequently, gram-negative bacteria are involved in acute suppurative parotitis [19]. Polycystic (dysgenetic) disease of the parotid glands is a very uncommon disorder that is not related to congenital sialectasis and recurrent parotitis [21]. Idiopathic recurrent pneumoparotitis is an infrequent disorder with painful swelling of the parotid gland and is also known as Wind Paroritis [22].

In terms of neoplasms, pleomorphic adenoma is a benign lesion that is the most common tumor of the salivary glands, mainly affecting the parotid serous gland [23]. Pleomorphic adenomas of the salivary gland are composed of luminal tumor cells and abluminal tumor cells [23, 24]. These cells form solid or proliferating structures inside the gland tissue and mesenchymal structures [24]. Pleomorphic adenoma usually involves the uppermost lobe of the parotid gland. This tumor is discussed in more detail in Section 9.9.

9.2 Mucous Salivary Gland

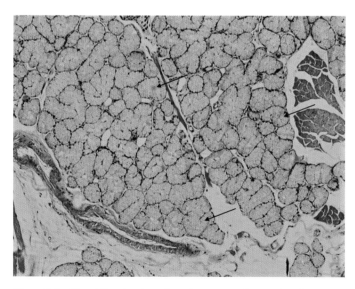

Figure 9.5 H and E stained section of mucous salivary gland (arrows, mucous acini).

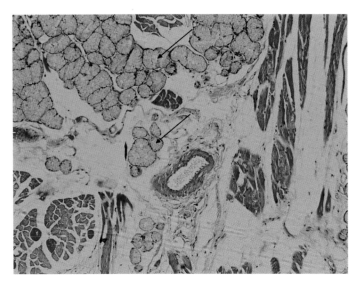

Figure 9.6 H and E stained section of mucous salivary gland (arrows, mucous acini).

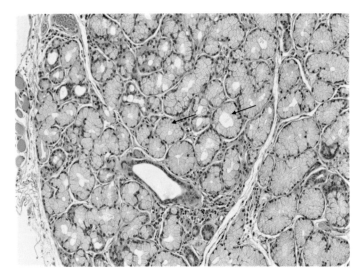

Figure 9.7 H and E stained section of mucous salivary gland (arrows, mucous acini).

9.2.1 Description

In the case of mucous salivary glands, a typical mucous cell has a tubular configuration with mucous surrounding a central lumen. The parotid or submandibular glands have a more significant number of intralobular ducts than the mucous salivary glands. Connective tissue septae divide different lobes of this gland. The mucous salivary gland cells have a large-sized Golgi complex present basal to the secretory granules. Due to the large size of the Golgi complex, the nucleus and rough endoplasmic reticulum are pressed against the basal cell membrane. Also, during the histologic preparations, the secretory aortas appear unstained or very lightly stained. Sublingual glands are one example of mucous salivary gland as they are composed primarily of mucous cells. Other example includes minor salivary glands.

9.2.2 Key Identifying Features

As the cells of this gland produce mucous, they do not stain darkly. The key feature of mucous cells is the accumulation of secretory mucus in the apical cytoplasm leading to an empty appearance of supranuclear cytoplasm.

9.2.3 Clinical Significance and Considerations

Mucin is secreted by these glands which acts as a lubricant in the saliva [5]. The mucous salivary gland contributes around 5% of the saliva which enters the oral cavity [1]. Ranulas are the most common pathologic lesion associated with the sublingual glands [25]. Ranulas and salivary gland retention cysts are commonly related to the group called tumor-like lesions. It can also be congenital or iatrogenic, maybe because of the trauma to the mouth and occlusion of salivary gland ducts. Damage to the ducts of minor and sublingual salivary glands may result in the extravasation of mucus into the surrounding soft tissues [25, 26]. Although not painful, larger-sized ranula may displace tongue, interfere with physiological swallowing, and cause dysphagia [26]. Clinically, ranulas present as intraoral or plunging ranulas. Plunging ranulas are a rare entity in which the salivary secretions spread into the soft tissues of the neck. When the pressure from the developing mucus, fluid enters through a gap in the mylohyoid muscle into the submandibular space, the plunging ranulas are formed.

In addition to ranula, other pathologies such as focal hyperplasia of minor salivary glands have been reported. First, Giansanti et al. reported in 1971 an asymptomatic palatal growth which was histologically characterized for proliferating mucous gland tissues [27]. Later, Devildos and Langlois reported minor salivary gland hyperplasia or adenoma originating from palatal glands [28]. Minor salivary glands' adenomatoid hyperplasia is not very common and histologically appears as aggregates of normal glandular cells. However, the clinical presentation of adenomatoid hyperplasia is like salivary gland neoplasms. The nature of such hyperplastic minor salivary gland lesions is complicated and not fully understood. Its presentation may range from simple hyperplasia to reactive hyperplasia or hamartoma [29].

9.3 Seromucous (Mixed) Salivary Gland

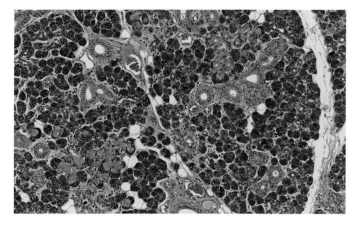

Figure 9.8 H and E stained section of mixed salivary gland with serous and mucous cells.

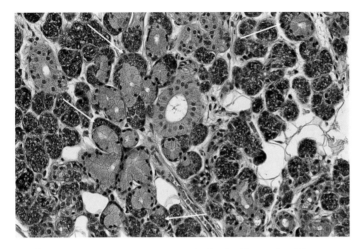

Figure 9.9 H and E stained section of mixed salivary gland (arrows, serous demilune).

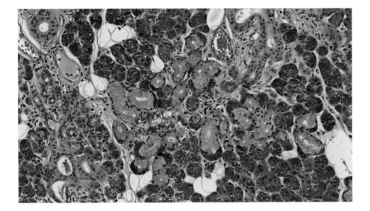

Figure 9.10 H and E stained section of seromucous gland with blood vessels and mixed cells.

9.3.1 Description

The mixed submandibular salivary glands are responsible to produce 65–70% of the saliva that enters the oral cavity, although they are much smaller in size as compared with the parotid gland. In addition to distinct serous and mucous areas, the formation of serous demilune is a prominent feature in this gland. The serous demilune is also known as Crescents of Giannuzzi or Demilunes of Heidenhain. These are the serous cells at the end of mucous secretory unit. The secretory units lead to intercalated ducts, the lining of which comprises simple low cuboidal epithelial cells surrounded by myoepithelial cells. The secretion of this type of gland is mixed (serous and mucous) and enters the oral cavity through Wharton's duct.

9.3.2 Key Identifying Features

The nuclei of serous cells are spherical and vesicular surrounded by pale staining granular cytoplasm. The nuclei of mucous cells are pushed against the basal cell membrane. Serous demilune, which are in the shape of half-moon, are clearly seen in this type of gland.

9.3.3 Clinical Significance and Considerations

The submandibular mixed salivary gland is essential to maintain bulk of the saliva produced. Its secretion can be disturbed due to various pathologies. Sialolith is a calcified stone and it frequently develops within the ductal system of the submandibular gland (Wharton's duct), possibly due to the submandibular duct's tortuous route toward its ductal opening [30, 31]. The development of calcific concretions in the major and minor salivary glands is known as Sialolithiasis [32]. Disturbed salivary secretion and microlithiasis lead to an increased bacterial load, which in turn causes degeneration of acinar cells and focal obstruction of acini. Increased deposition of calcium and phosphate salts is another cause of sialolith formation, which causes accumulation of desquamated cells, along with the bacteria and salivary mucus. Salivary dysfunction, infections, ductal anomalies, and ductal epithelium metaplasia are also considered to be the possible cause of sialolith formation [33]. Sialoliths are more common in males than women and middle-aged disease. The clinical representation of the sialoliths is swelling and pain in the damaged part of the glands [30, 32].

9.4 Intercalated Ducts

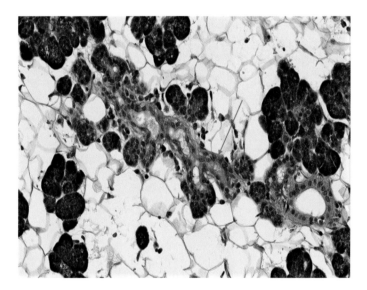

Figure 9.11 H and E stained section of serous gland (arrow, intercalated duct).

9.4.1 Description

The intercalated ducts have a lining of simple cuboidal epithelium. The nuclei in the duct cells appear prominent, owing to the relatively scanty cytoplasm. In addition, bodies and processes of myoepithelial cells are typically positioned alongside the duct's basal surface.

9.4.2 Key Identifying Features

Intercalated ducts are characteristically long, narrow, and branching. Several intercalated ducts are seen converging toward the center of the field. Clusters of serous secretory acini can be seen at the ends of the two intercalated ducts.

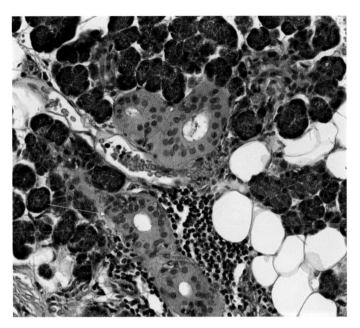

Figure 9.12 H and E stained section of serous gland (arrow, intercalated duct).

9.4.3 Clinical Significance and Considerations

These intercalated ducts lead the salivary secretion from acinus toward striated duct. Salivary glands intercalated duct may have rare tumors due to pathological proliferation of the duct cells, ranging from hyperplasia to adenoma in terms of a morphologic spectrum. The pathological proliferation of the intercalated ducts may ensue due to several reasons, including chronic sialadenitis [34, 35].

9.5 Striated Ducts

9.5.1 Description

Striated ducts are formed by the union of intercalated ducts. The columnar cells of the striated ducts have a large amount of pale, acidophilic cytoplasm and a large, spherical, centrally positioned nucleus. The primary saliva drains to the striated ducts from the intercalated ducts. The basal cytoplasm of the duct cells shows deep folding and produces sheet-like folds. These folds extend to the lateral boundaries of the cells and then link with the folds of the adjacent cells.

9.5.2 Key Identifying Features

On histological sections, these ducts appear with striations as the basal cytoplasm is striated. The cells of the striated duct are highly polarized. Their luminal surfaces have short microvilli. The striated ducts are the key locations for electrolytes' resorption (such as sodium and chloride) and secretion (such as potassium and bicarbonate) without the loss of water.

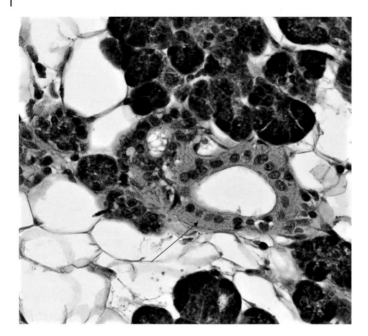

Figure 9.13 H and E stained section of serous gland (arrow, striated duct).

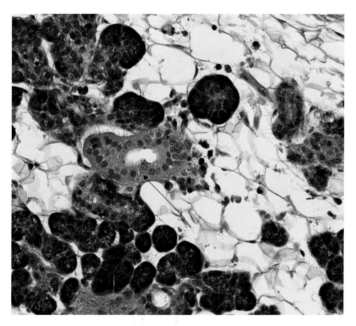

Figure 9.14 H and E stained section of serous gland (arrow, striated duct).

9.5.3 Clinical Significance and Considerations

The striated ducts represent a highly infolded plasma membrane with mitochondria in the cytoplasm between the folds at the cells' base. The Na^+ and Cl^- ions from the primary secretion are reabsorbed by striated ducts and their folded cell membranes. This facilitates the rapid ion transportation and modifies salivary fluid by secreting $HCO3^-$ and K^+, therefore, helping in the hypotonicity of the secretion. Striated duct adenoma (SDA) of the salivary gland is an unusual benign tumor which is present mainly in the parotid glands [36]. It is unilayered encapsulated tumor that recapitulates normal striated ducts. This type of tumor has distinctive features of eosinophilic cytoplasm with hypervascular stroma and papillary thyroid carcinoma-like nuclei [37]. Among unilayered salivary gland tumors, canalicular adenoma (CA) is the tumor most comparable to SDA. A CA is the only recognized tumor with pure luminal cell differentiation. CA tumors are characterized histologically by cystic spaces, tumor cords with beading tubule formation, eosinophilic cytoplasm without striations, a myxoid stroma, luminal balls, hemorrhages, and microliths [38, 39].

9.6   Excretory Ducts

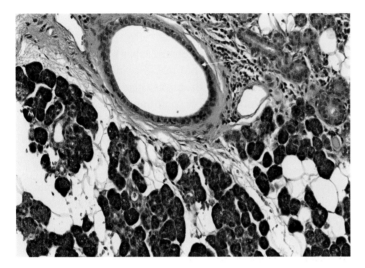

Figure 9.15   H and E stained section of serous gland (arrow, excretory duct).

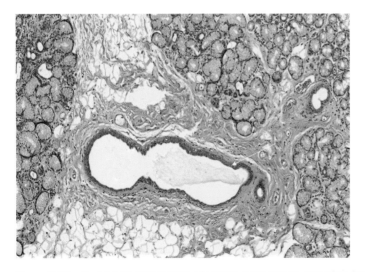

Figure 9.16   H and E stained section of serous gland (arrow, excretory duct).

9.6.1 Description

The excretory ducts are lined by pseudostratified columnar epithelium and pass through the connective tissue septae between the salivary tissue lobules. Its epithelial lining may change to stratified type near the oral opening. A large excretory duct is surrounded by dense connective tissues. The pseudostratified epithelium contains several mucous goblet cells.

9.6.2 Key Identifying Features

The presence of tuft or brush cells with long stiff microvilli is considered as receptor cells due to the existence of the nerve ending close to the basal portion of cells. The interlobular artery supplies the interlobular excretory ducts through a subepithelial network of capillaries and drains into the interlobular vein. This forms the intralobular circulation different from the excretory duct circulation.

9.6.3 Clinical Significance and Considerations

As their name suggests, the function of excretory ducts is to excrete the saliva in oral cavity. These excretory ducts belonging to different salivary glands open in the oral cavity in different locations. The excretory duct reserve cell may be the origination point of salivary gland tumors with squamous or mucinous cell differentiation. A common inflammatory condition called infectious parotitis or mumps usually affects children till the age of 15 years [40]. There is distention of small intraparenchymal excretory ducts. Also, there is an occurrence of abnormal dilatation of the duct usually congenital or acquired [41]. Secondary inflammation results from the stasis of the secretions. Strictures and stenosis cause decreased salivary flow which in turn causes change to the excretory duct epithelium of the salivary gland with metaplasia. Mucous secretion is produced abundantly due to the metaplasia of the duct epithelium. Typical duct ectasia is caused due to the weakened surrounding connective tissue. The excretory duct reserve cells may originate salivary gland tumors with squamous or mucinous cell differentiation.

9.7 Sialadenitis

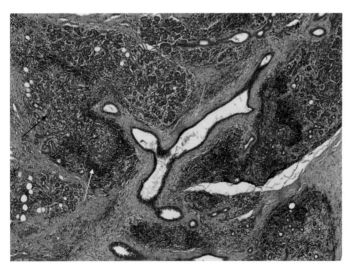

Figure 9.17 H and E stained section of serous gland (white arrow, inflammatory cells; black arrow, damaged acini; orange arrow, fibrosis).

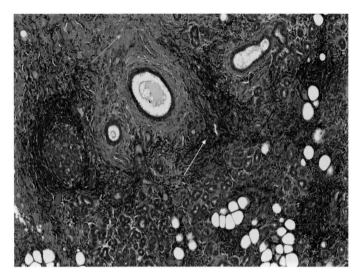

Figure 9.18 H and E stained section of serous gland (white arrow, inflammatory cells; black arrow, damaged acini; orange arrow, fibrosis).

9.7.1 Description

Sialadenitis signifies parotid, submandibular, sublingual, or minor salivary gland inflammation and swelling. Etiology covers bacterial or viral infection, blockage, or autoimmune diseases. Acute bacterial sialadenitis is characterized by pain and swelling at a rapid onset. Chronic sialadenitis, by contrast, is characterized by sporadic, recurring bouts of tender swelling. In terms of pathogens that cause sialadenitis, the viruses are far more common than bacteria. Mumps is the most common of viral causes that affect either the parotid (more common) or the submandibular gland, but other viral causes include Coxsackie, parainfluenza, and HIV. The pain, tenderness, redness, and graduated localized swelling of the affected zone can be associated with a sialadenitis. Elderly and chronically ill people with a dry mouth or with dehydration suffer most from sialadenitis.

9.7.2 Key Identifying Features

The related histological specimen illustrates substantial fibrosis, chronic inflammation, acinar atrophy, and ductal residual elements.

9.7.3 Clinical Considerations

Different modalities of imaging are crucial for the diagnosis of sialadenitis. The association of imaging results with the clinical presentation and laboratory testing helps to determine the precise cause of sialadenitis and aids the clinician to choose the appropriate mode of treatment. With hydration and analgesia, most patients are treated conservatively. For situations where saliva production is compromised, artificial saliva may be used [42]. If bacterial sialadenitis is doubted, antibiotics should be administered. Patients with persistent sialadenitis may benefit from surgical gland removal. Extreme cases can lead to abscess development, which can lead to obstruction of the airway that is considered a medical emergency [43].

9.8 Necrotizing Sialometaplasia

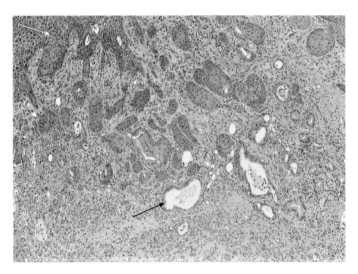

Figure 9.19 H and E stained section of necrotizing sialometaplasia (white arrow, pseudoepitheliomatous hyperplasia of surface epithelium; black arrow, squamous metaplasia in salivary ducts).

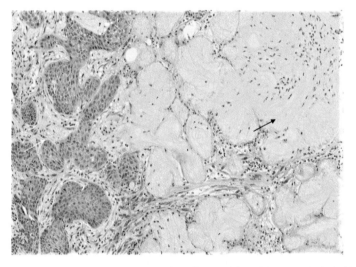

Figure 9.20 H and E stained section of necrotizing sialometaplasia (white arrow, squamous metaplasia in salivary ducts; black arrow, necrotic acini with a "Ghost-like" appearance).

9.8.1 Description

Necrotizing sialometaplasia is a self-restricting benign inflammatory reaction of salivary gland tissue that can resemble squamous cell carcinoma or mucoepidermoid carcinoma. It shows squamous metaplasia of salivary gland ducts, necrosis of the acini with prominent pseudoepitheliomatous hyperplasia of the surface epithelium most commonly involving the hard palate.

Despite the worrisome appearance, there is no evidence of dysplasia or mitotic figures which can help to differentiate it from a malignancy. The pathogenesis is ambiguous, but it is assumed to be because of vasculature ischemia that supplies the lobules of the salivary gland. There are several factors that cause ischemia, such as direct trauma, local anesthetic administration, defective dentures, etc. The minor salivary glands in the palate are the most frequently affected site. Many other locations, such as retromolar pad, gingiva, ear, tongue, nose, nasal cavity, sinuses, larynx, and trachea where the tissue of the salivary gland is positioned may also be involved. The lesion is generally painful and, often 1–3 cm in diameter, and is described as a well-circumscribed ulcer.

9.8.2 Key Identifying Features

The overall preservation of lobular architecture is the primary characteristic histopathologic trait of necrotizing sialometaplasia. Pseudoepitheliomatous hyperplasia and ductal squamous metaplasia and acini are other diagnostic features.

9.8.3 Clinical Considerations

Diagnosis of necrotizing sialometaplasia is complex and is dependent on a full clinical history and well-conducted biopsy [44]. The most representative sample is provided by biopsy taken from the base of the ulcer and the edge which is most indurated and raised and clinically resembles a squamous cell carcinoma. An amalgamation of histopathological and clinical findings is often supportive when arriving at a confirmatory diagnosis. No treatment is normally essential and the lesion heals within 4–10 weeks by secondary intention [45].

9.9 Pleomorphic Adenoma

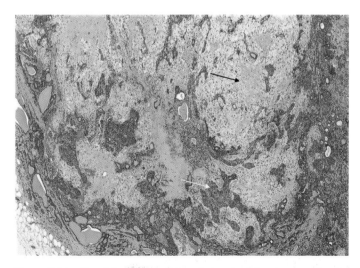

Figure 9.21 H and E stained section of pleomorphic adenoma showing a variety of appearances (white arrow, epithelial cells; black arrow, stroma).

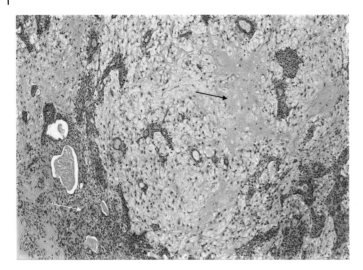

Figure 9.22 H and E stained section of pleomorphic adenoma showing a variety of appearances (white arrow, epithelial cells; black arrow, stroma; orange arrow, duct).

9.9.1 Description

Pleomorphic adenoma is also recognized as a mixed benign tumor because it originates from epithelial and myoepithelial elements, and is the most common type of salivary gland tumor. It accounts for up to two-thirds of all salivary gland tumors. The most frequently involved salivary gland is the parotid gland. Among the minor salivary glands locations, the palate is most frequently involved site followed by lips, cheeks, gingiva, the floor of the mouth, and tongue. Pleomorphic adenoma presents mostly as a slowly growing, painless, solitary mobile mass, which may have been present for several years.

9.9.2 Key Identifying Features

Microscopically, pleomorphic adenoma has a highly variable appearance, hence the name pleomorphic. It is described as a mixed proliferation of polygonal epithelial and spindle-shaped or plasmacytoid myoepithelial cells in a variable stroma matrix of mucoid, myxoid, cartilaginous, or hyaline origin. Epithelial components typically consist of polygonal, spindle, or stellate-shaped cells that can be organized to form duct-like structures, sheets, clumps, or strands that interlace. Apart from an inner cuboidal epithelial cell layer, the ducts and acini are normally seen showing an outer lining. Presence of squamous metaplasia and tyrosine crystals (within ducts) can also be useful identifying features.

9.9.3 Clinical Considerations

The diagnosis of this condition is histological. Procedures for the diagnosis through tissue sampling include fine-needle aspiration (FNA) and the core needle biopsy. The variation in appearance within a tumor can make diagnosis challenging on limited tissue and small biopsies. The ideal treatment for pleomorphic adenomas is surgical excision [46]. Even though the lesion is benign, there is a reported recurrence rate of 8–45% [47]. Some long-standing pleomorphic adenomas can undergo malignant change resulting in a carcinoma ex pleomorphic adenoma (CexPA). The patient usually presents with a history of a long-standing lesion but with recent increase in size or appearance of symptoms [48]. The common signs and symptoms of CexPA include pain, swelling, paraesthesia, and ulceration of the overlying mucosa/skin [49]. The diagnosis of CexPA is mainly histological and treatment commonly involves the use of trastuzumab (anticancer drug) and radiotherapy [50].

9.10 Warthin Tumor

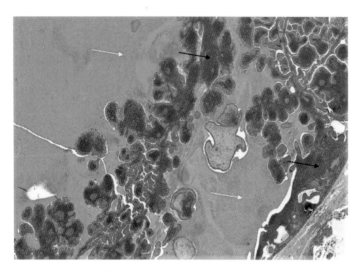

Figure 9.23 H and E stained section of a Warthin tumor (white arrows, cystic areas; black arrows, lymphoid tissue in stroma).

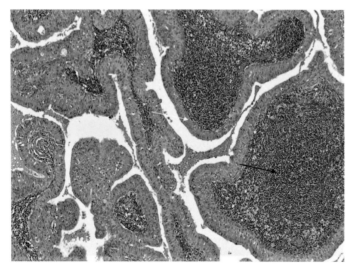

Figure 9.24 H and E stained section of a Warthin tumor (white arrow, oncocytic epithelium lining the cystic areas; black arrow, lymphoid tissue in stroma).

9.10.1 Description

Warthin tumor is a benign cystic salivary gland tumor that contains abundant lymphocytes and germinal centers (stroma which is like a lymph node). Warthin tumor's other name, papillary cystadenoma lymphomatosum, is long and technical but describes the disease well whereas adenolymphoma is now considered incorrect. Parotid gland is the most likely involved salivary gland. It is the only tumor that is virtually confined to the parotid gland and the second-most common benign tumor of the parotid gland. Occasional cases of minor salivary gland involvement have been reported [51–53]. Warthin tumor is typically slow-growing and it can take years before symptoms appear – which usually involve a painless slow-growing swelling.

9.10.2   Key Identifying Features

Microscopically, two components are seen in Warthin tumor, epithelial and lymphoid. As the name papillary cystadenoma lymphomatosum indicates, this lesion is cystic, with papillary processes lined by oncocytic epithelium, projecting into the cystic space. The surrounding connective tissue has abundant lymphoid components exhibiting germinal centers. The epithelium lining the papillary projections is bilayered with inner cuboidal cells and outer columnar cells. Columnar cells are regularly arranged to have a palisading arrangement of nuclei. Cystic space usually contains eosinophilic secretory material.

9.10.3   Clinical Considerations

Parotidectomy is the standard surgical treatment. Capsular dissection without formal parotidectomy is a reasonable alternative in selected cases due to the benign, non-recurrent nature of the tumor [54].

References

1 Khurshid, Z., Naseem, M., Sheikh, Z. et al. (2016). Oral antimicrobial peptides: types and role in the oral cavity. *Saudi Pharm J* 24 (5): 515–524.

2 Holmberg, K.V. and Hoffman, M.P. (2014). Anatomy, biogenesis and regeneration of salivary glands. *Monogr Oral Sci* 24: 1–13.

3 Khurshid, Z., Zafar, M.S., Khan, R.S. et al. (2018). Role of salivary biomarkers in oral cancer detection. *Adv Clin Chem* 86: 23–70.

4 Tiwari, M. (2011). Science behind human saliva. *J Nat Sci Biol Med* 2 (1): 53–58.

5 Khurshid, Z., Zohaib, S., Najeeb, S. et al. (2016). Human saliva collection devices for proteomics: an update. *Int J Mol Sci* 17 (6): 846.

6 Dawes, C., Pedersen, A.M., Villa, A. et al. (2015). The functions of human saliva: a review sponsored by the World Workshop on Oral Medicine VI. *Arch Oral Biol* 60 (6): 863–874.

7 Khurshid, Z., Mali, M., Naseem, M. et al. (2017). Human gingival crevicular fluids (GCF) proteomics: an overview. *Dent J (Basel)* 5 (1): 12.

8 Khurshid, Z. (2018). Salivary point-of-care technology. *Eur J Dent* 12(1): 1–2.

9 Khurshid, Z., Zafar, M.S., Naseem, M. et al. (2018). Human oral defensins antimicrobial peptides: a future promising antimicrobial drug. *Curr Pharm Des* 24 (10): 1130–1137.

10 Khurshid, Z., Najeeb, S., Mali, M. et al. (2017). Histatin peptides: pharmacological functions and their applications in dentistry. *Saudi Pharm J* 25 (1): 25–31.

11 Khurshid, Z., Naseem, M., Yahya, I. et al. (2017). Significance and diagnostic role of antimicrobial cathelicidins (LL-37) peptides in oral health. *Biomolecules* 7 (4): 80.

12 Abdul Rehman, S., Khurshid, Z., Hussain Niazi, F. et al. (2017). Role of salivary biomarkers in detection of cardiovascular diseases (CVD). *Proteomes* 5 (3): 21.

13 Sannam Khan, R., Khurshid, Z., Akhbar, S., and Faraz Moin, S. (2016). Advances of salivary proteomics in oral squamous cell carcinoma (OSCC) detection: an update. *Proteomes* 4 (4): 41.

14 Sahibzada, H.A., Khurshid, Z., Khan, R.S. et al. (2017). Salivary IL-8, IL-6 and TNF-α as potential diagnostic biomarkers for oral cancer. *Diagnostics (Basel)* 7 (2): 21.

15 Khurshid, Z., Asiri, F.Y.I., and Al Wadaani, H. (2020). Human saliva: non-invasive fluid for detecting novel coronavirus (2019-nCoV). *Int J Environ Res Public Health* 17 (7): 2225.

16 Corstjens, P.L., Abrams, W.R., and Malamud, D. (2012). Detecting viruses by using salivary diagnostics. *J Am Dent Assoc* 143 (10 Suppl): 12S–18S.

17 Khurshid, Z., Zafar, M., Khan, E. et al. (2019). Human saliva can be a diagnostic tool for Zika virus detection. *J Infect Public Health* 12 (5): 601–604.

18 Porcheri, C. and Mitsiadis, T.A. (2019). Physiology, pathology and regeneration of salivary glands. *Cells* 8 (9): 976.

19 Brook, I. (1992). Diagnosis and management of parotitis. *Arch Otolaryngol Head Neck Surg* 118 (5): 469–471.

20 Patel, P., Scott, S., and Cunningham, S. (2017). Challenging case of parotitis: a comprehensive approach. *J Am Osteopath Assoc* 117 (12): e137–e140.

21 Seifert, G., Thomsen, S., and Donath, K. (1981). Bilateral dysgenetic polycystic parotid glands. Morphological analysis and differential diagnosis of a rare disease of the salivary glands. *Virchows Arch A Pathol Anat Histol* 390 (3): 273–288.

22 McCormick, M.E., Bawa, G., and Shah, R.K. (2013). Idiopathic recurrent pneumoparotitis. *Am J Otolaryngol* 34 (2): 180–182.

23 Ogawa, Y., Kishino, M., Atsumi, Y. et al. (2003). Plasmacytoid cells in salivary-gland pleomorphic adenomas: evidence of luminal cell differentiation. *Virchows Arch* 443 (5): 625–634.

24 Sreeja, C., Shahela, T., Aesha, S., and Satish, M.K. (2014). Taxonomy of salivary gland neoplasm. *J Clin Diagn Res* 8 (3): 291–293.

25 Sheikhi, M., Jalalian, F., Rashidipoor, R., and Mosavat, F. (2011). Plunging ranula of the submandibular area. *Dent Res J (Isfahan)* 8 (Suppl 1): S114–S118.

26 de Visscher, J.G., van der Wal, K.G., and de Vogel, P.L. (1989). The plunging ranula. Pathogenesis, diagnosis and management. *J Craniomaxillofac Surg* 17 (4): 182–185.

27 Giansanti, J.S., Baker, G.O., and Waldron, C.A. (1971). Intraoral, mucinous, minor salivary gland lesions presenting clinically as tumors. *Oral Surg Oral Med Oral Pathol* 32 (6): 918–922.

28 Devildos, L.R. and Langlois, C.C. (1976). Minor salivary gland lesion presenting clinically as tumor. *Oral Surg Oral Med Oral Pathol* 41 (5): 657–659.

29 Buchner, A., Merrell, P.W., Carpenter, W.M., and Leider, A.S. (1991). Adenomatoid hyperplasia of minor salivary glands. *Oral Surg Oral Med Oral Pathol* 71 (5): 583–587.

30 Alkurt, M.T. and Peker, I. (2009). Unusually large submandibular sialoliths: report of two cases. *Eur J Dent* 3 (2): 135–139.

31 Shahoon, H., Farhadi, S., and Hamedi, R. (2015). Giant sialoliths of Wharton duct: report of two rare cases and review of literature. *Dent Res J (Isfahan)* 12 (5): 494–497.

32 Huang, T.C., Dalton, J.B., Monsour, F.N., and Savage, N.W. (2009). Multiple, large sialoliths of the submandibular gland duct: a case report. *Aust Dent J* 54 (1): 61–65.

33 Arifa, S.P., Christopher, P.J., Kumar, S. et al. (2019). Sialolithiasis of the submandibular gland: report of cases. *Cureus* 11 (3): e4180.

34 Yu, G.Y. and Donath, K. (2001). Adenomatous ductal proliferation of the salivary gland. *Oral Surg Oral Med Oral Pathol Oral Radiol Endod* 91 (2): 215–221.

35 Naunheim, M.R., Lin, H.W., Faquin, W.C., and Lin, D.T. (2012). Intercalated duct lesion of the parotid. *Head Neck Pathol* 6 (3): 373–376.

36 Weinreb, I., Simpson, R.H., Skálová, A. et al. (2010). Ductal adenomas of salivary gland showing features of striated duct differentiation ('striated duct adenoma'): a report of six cases. *Histopathology* 57 (5): 707–715.

37 Ito, Y., Fujii, K., Murase, T. et al. (2017). Striated duct adenoma presenting with intra-tumoral hematoma and papillary thyroid carcinoma-like histology. *Pathol Int* 67 (6): 316–321.

38 Thompson, L.D., Bauer, J.L., Chiosea, S. et al. (2015). Canalicular adenoma: a clinicopathologic and immunohistochemical analysis of 67 cases with a review of the literature. *Head Neck Pathol* 9 (2): 181–195.

39 Weinreb, I., Seethala, R.R., Hunt, J.L. et al. (2009). Intercalated duct lesions of salivary gland: a morphologic spectrum from hyperplasia to adenoma. *Am J Surg Pathol* 33 (9): 1322–1329.

40 Zenk, J., Schneider, H., Koch, M. et al. (2014). Current management of juvenile recurrent parotitis. *Curr Otorhinolaryngol Rep* 2: 64–69.

41 Toft-Nielsen, C., Howitz, M.F., Glenthøj, J., and Foghsgaard, J. (2019). Salivary gland diseases in children. *Ugeskr Laeger* 181 (22): V1180819.

42 Madani, G. and Beale, T. (2006). Inflammatory conditions of the salivary glands. *Semin Ultrasound CT MRI* 27: 440–451.

43 Ugga, L., Ravanelli, M., Pallottino, A.A. et al. (2017). Diagnostic work-up in obstructive and inflammatory salivary gland disorders. Work-up diagnostico nella patologia ostruttiva e infiammatoria delle ghiandole salivari. *Acta Otorhinolaryngol Ital* 37 (2): 83–93.

44 Ramagosa, V., Bella, M.R., Truchero, C., and Moya, J. (1992). Necrotizing sialometaplasia (adenometaplasia) of the trachea. *Histopathology* 21 (3): 280–282.

45 Joshi, S.A., Halli, R., Koranne, V., and Singh, S. (2014). Necrotizing sialometaplasia: a diagnostic dilemma. *J Oral Maxillofac Pathol* 18 (3): 420–422.

46 Valentini, V., Fabiani, F., Perugini, M. et al. (2001). Surgical techniques in the treatment of pleomorphic adenoma of the parotid gland: our experience and review of literature. *J Craniofac Surg* 12 (6): 565–568.

47 Park, S.Y., Han, K.T., Kim, M.C., and Lim, J.S. (2016). Recurrent pleomorphic adenoma of the parotid gland. *Arch Craniofac Surg* 17 (2): 90–92.

48 Di Palma, S. (2013). Carcinoma ex pleomorphic adenoma, with particular emphasis on early lesions. *Head Neck Pathol* 7 (Suppl 1(Suppl 1)): S68–S76.

49 Tamgadge, S., Tamgadge, A., Pereira, T., and Naik, S. (2014). Carcinoma ex pleomorphic adenoma: rare malignant salivary gland neoplasm. *Oral Hyg Health* 2: 133.

50 Sharon, E., Kelly, R.J., and Szabo, E. (2010). Sustained response of carcinoma ex pleomorphic adenoma treated with trastuzumab and capecitabine. *Head Neck Oncol* 2: 12.

51 Diaz-Segarra, N., Young, L.K., Levin, K. et al. (2018). Warthin tumor of the oropharyngeal minor salivary gland. *SAGE Open Med Case Rep* 6: 2050313X18818712.

52 Iwai, T., Baba, J., Murata, S. et al. (2012). Warthin tumor arising from the minor salivary gland. *J Craniofac Surg* 23 (5): e374–e376.

53 Gao, Z., Aladimi, M.T., Xuan, M. et al. (2017). An unusual Warthin's tumor arising from minor salivary glands in the floor of mouth. *Int J Clin Exp Med* 10 (5): 8385–8388.

54 Chulam, T.C., Noronha Francisco, A.L., Goncalves Filho, J. et al. (2013). Warthin's tumour of the parotid gland: our experience. *Acta Otorhinolaryngol Ital* 33 (6): 393–397.

Index

Page numbers in *italics* refer to illustrations; those in **bold** refer to tables

An Illustrated Guide to Oral Histology, First Edition. Edited by Imran Farooq, Saqib Ali, and Paul Anderson.
© 2021 John Wiley & Sons Ltd. Published 2021 by John Wiley & Sons Ltd.
Companion website: www.wiley.com/go/farooq/oral_histology